MENIER

AND THE ASTRONAUT

THE
SELF HELP
BOOK
FOR
MENIERE'S
DISEASE

Contents

Meniere Man And The Astronaut 5
Why Meniere's 11
What Is Meniere's Disease 15
Diagnosis Of Meniere's Disease 17
The Benefits Of Tinnitus 23
Meniere's At Work 25
Meniere's At Home 29
Time And Money Matters 31
The Pharmacy 35
Surgical Options 39
What Causes Meniere's Disease 43
Doing Life With Meniere's Disease 45
Triggers For Meniere's Attacks 51
Avoiding Stress Overload 57
Mechanics Of An Attack 61
Spinning Out 63
How To Cope During An Attack 67
Why Meniere's Affects Hearing 69
The Emotional Effect Of Hearing Loss 75
The Well-Being Scale 81
Cognitive Issues 85
Meniere's Circles 87
Burning Out Of Meniere's 89
Meniere's Management 91
Eat. Drink. Play. 105
Environmental Equations 113
Alternative Therapies 115
A Strategy For Wellness 127
Talk To Yourself 131
The Hi Friend 133
Laugh. Love. Live. 135
Postscript 137
One Hundred Ways Of Coping With Meniere's 140
Books By Meniere Man 147
Meniere's Support Networks And Societies 148
Books Meniere Man Recommends 150
About Meniere Man 151
Additional Information 154

Meniere Man
And The
Astronaut

If you have been diagnosed with Meniere's disease, you are in good company. There have been many famous Meniere sufferers, such as Alan Shepard the astronaut, Vincent Van Gogh the artist, Jonathan Swift author, Peggy Lee singer, Martin Luther human rights leader, Emily Dickenson author, Tim Conley professional golfer, and of course, yours truly!

In *The Self Help Book For Meniere's Disease*, I have written down specific aspects relevant to Meniere's sufferers based on my personal experience of having had the disease.

To give you a brief background, when I was diagnosed with Meniere's disease, I was forty-six. A fit man at the height of his professional career;

running his own business, married, with a young family of two.

Not only was it devastating news, it was extremely difficult to know what to do or how to cope, because I was given no real answers about Meniere's disease.

While relatively easy to diagnose, medical professionals don't agree on the prognosis and outcome of Meniere's disease. This makes it difficult for the patient to put a successful management plan in place.

At the time of my diagnosis there was little information about the disease or how to manage the symptoms. There were no books on the subject. So I had no idea what to expect or how to effectively manage the condition. What I did know was the acute attacks of vertigo were breaking my spirit. As well as trying to cope with vertigo attacks, the loss of life's equilibrium, gave me an increasing worry about where Meniere's disease was taking me and my family.

For the first time in my life, I felt a constant sense of anxiety and fear. I was at a complete loss. The specialists and doctors couldn't give me comprehensive and definitive answers on how to manage the condition.

So how would I cope and get well again? I decided to take responsibility for figuring out how to overcome this condition and make a new life. Working through the condition from illness to wellness has enabled me to write this book and other books in the Meniere Man series.

Meniere's has had a massive impact on my life; my successful business career has gone, but these days I am symptom free and I have a positive outlook on the future. There is a saying, "It takes one to know one." Unlike a medical text, this book is from the point-of-view of someone who has been there and knows the boundaries of this disease. I understand what you are going through. I have been in the depths of despair. In my mind, I associate Meniere's with some of the most frightening experiences of my life.

The out-of-control nature of Meniere's attacks creates emotional, mental, social and physical uncertainty. But despite your diagnosis, you will be able, through determination and effort, to regain a sense of power and equilibrium in your life.

As human beings, we need to have a sense of control over our activities and confidence in where we are going. Meniere's takes this away from you. Not being in control creates an unnerving feeling and not being able to find answers seems to exasperate how we feel. The more anxious we get, the worse we feel.

We can get lost in the symptoms of disease, but having the right information can act as a map back to our sense of inherent well-being. In times of serious illness, we need hope and a belief in a positive outcome. This is what gives us the strength to overcome the disabling affects of the disease.

I not only understand the devastating effects of having Meniere's disease, but how Meniere's can have a beneficial impact. Meniere's makes you listen to your body intently; which enables you to find ways to greatly improve your overall physical and psychological health. You can end up in a better state of health and well-being than before you were diagnosed with Meniere's.

By sharing what has worked for me, my hope is that you will be able to re-construct your own life as quickly as possible. In a short time, you will be able to do the seemingly impossible.

When I was having acute Meniere's attacks, I couldn't look up without going dizzy. I couldn't tie my shoelaces without feeling woozy. I never imagined I would get back to normal; let alone learn to snowboard and windsurf while I was suffering the symptoms of Meniere's. Yet it was these balancing activities that helped me regain my equilibrium.

The more you do, the better you feel. The more you try, the more you achieve. It is one step at a time on the road to recovery. Until eventually it will be you going on long hikes through mountainous terrain. It will be you completely well again. Meniere's will be behind you.

The only reminder I have of ever having the

disease is hearing loss in one ear and Tinnitus. You won't hear me complain about that physical detail. I am grateful for what I have. In short, I have a full life again.

Why Meniere's

The Medical profession has been trying since 1861 to find the cause and cure for Meniere's disease. But Meniere's has proven to be an elusive condition to cure. However the effect on the Meniere's sufferer is anything but elusive; it is a very confrontational and challenging disease. When I was diagnosed with Meniere's disease in 1995 I found very little information on the day to day, hour to hour management of Meniere's. What didn't elude me was the impact Meniere's was having on my life; but there was more to come.

Tinnitus (ringing in the ear) is a side effect of Meniere's disease and it can be a constant challenge. Over the years, the noises changed as my brain adapted to the condition...but the first experience, was the most frightening event of my life, the sound was inside my head and I couldn't turn it off. It sounded like I was traveling inside a 747 airliner day and night; the cabin filled with cicadas amid the constant roar of the jet engines with no respite.

Meniere's with its vertigo attacks and associated Tinnitus was hard to cope with. My days were full of fear. At times, I was afraid to open my eyes and start another day. A slight movement of my head on the pillow, or turning over in the early hours of the morning, gave me a dizzy sick feeling. Another day, a repeat of the day before and the weeks before that. The fear of spontaneous spinning. The fear of not being able to communicate effectively. Fear of being unable to concentrate. This turned into financial fear. Fear of failing in my business. Fear of family disruption, of people thinking less of me. Social fear. Being afraid to go to the movies in case I spun out in public.

I had trouble hearing what people were saying. I must have appeared vague, staring blankly as if disinterested. Yawning and tired. Even my family lost patience. They couldn't understand how I was feeling and just wanted me to be my 'old self'.

Within months, I knew I was failing in my business. The random nature of attacks, meant I would suddenly start to spin in a meeting with clients. The post production after hours, in small studios with artificial lighting, often caused me to excuse myself and have another director take over. I was running out of excuses.

I knew I couldn't continue in my business with the stress, the overwhelming exhaustion and acute Meniere's attacks. I was a key member of the business and I felt embarrassed and threatened by what was happening. Clients' and staff relied on me to make right decisions. The competitive nature of the business meant that other agencies were always hunting our business.

In that competitive environment, I was aware I was the sick one. The weakest link. Yet my pride would not let me admit to the office, my business partners and clients, that I now had an incurable disease and the symptoms were causing me to fail. Unable to work at my job, and with no understanding as to when I would be cured. I knew I would have to leave the company with as little disruption to the business as possible. This is exactly what I did.

I left the business at the height of my professional career and existed for a while on a Income Protection Plan. Three years later, the insurers cancelled my claim. We then lost all family assets to lawyers and the insurance company.

In so many ways, the diagnosis of Meniere's disease changed my life dramatically. It is not just the physical nature of the disease, as it affects the body, but how it affects people around you as well. Family, friends and unfortunately for some, fortunes and a secure financial future.

Looking back, I would place emphasis on not relying on others to understand the medical condition. The lesson I take from my experience is to seek empathetic, altruistic people to help you and your family through this. To be as self-reliant as you can in financial matters.

What Is Meniere's Disease

Meniere's was identified as a condition in 1861 by a French physician by the name of Prosper Meniere. It's a fancy name for a fearful condition. My understanding is this. Meniere's is an idiopathic syndrome of endolymphatic hydrops. This is the medical definition: Idiopathic means; unknown cause. Endolymphatic, refers to endolymph, a fluid in the inner ear. Hydrops means excessive fluid build-up. When you put it all together - idiopathic endolymphatic hydrops means; the unknown cause of excessive endolymphatic fluid build up in the inner ear. This build up of fluid and its consequent flooding effect is what causes the symptoms of vertigo, Tinnitus and progressive deafness.

The condition with all its vertigo, vomiting and spinning, is still not totally understood by specialists today. I have had Meniere's described to me by doctors as an incurable disease which has no known cause or origin. The underlying cause of Meniere disease can only be speculative. Meniere's disease is unpredictable which makes diagnosis and management extremely difficult.

Every person with Meniere's has a different cascade of symptoms and effects, although there are main symptoms, there is an infinite variety of presentations and timing. Some specialists however say they can cure or eradicate the symptoms. I was not convinced and in my case, I managed the symptoms without surgery.

Diagnosis Of Meniere's Disease

Meniere's can only be identified, with certainty, after death by histopathologic study of the temporal bones. Fortunately, it can also be diagnosed while you are alive by identifying, spontaneous episodic vertigo attacks, measurable hearing loss, aural fullness and Tinnitus. These are the internationally accepted criteria for a Meniere's disease diagnosis.

For a doctor to diagnose Meniere's, you have had at least two definite rotational vertigo attacks of twenty minutes or longer. Rotational means the spinning goes around as though you have a weight on the end of a rope and you are spinning around and around horizontally. Vertigo is the sensation of movement when no movement is taking place.

Vertigo

Vertigo, the spinning movement, usually makes you feel nauseous to a point of vomiting or retching. However, you do not and will not lose consciousness. During the attack of vertigo, horizontal rotary nystagmus is always active (the eyes involuntarily flicking from side to side). This type of vertigo is termed episodic vertigo of the Meniere's type.

Hearing Loss

Even without testing, you know your own body. In everyday situations you'll notice your hearing has dropped. This may only be an impression as your Tinnitus or aural fullness can make it feel like you have lost hearing. How much you think you have lost will be subjective, so hearing loss has to be documented.

Depending on what specialist you are seeing the specific technical recordings of your hearing loss will be decided by your specialist. Typically, the hearing loss is in the lower frequencies. So, you will be having difficulty understanding what people are saying, and missing fragments of conversation, especially if there is background sound like kitchen clatter, music, television or air conditioning.

Hearing loss is determined by an examination in an audio clinic. Your hearing may or may not fluctuate in the early stages of Meniere's disease. Typically it does in the early stages, but your hearing loss has to be documented by an audio-metric test to satisfy the criteria set by your ENT (ear, nose and throat) Specialist. The specific loss has to be identified in the affected ear, at least on one occasion by an audio metric test.

Aural Fullness

Aural fullness feels like having a soft wad of damp cotton wool inside the ear, blocking sound out. This sensation of fullness is the fluid pressure building up in the inner ear. The symptom of Aural fullness can be a useful marker for you. It can signal that a vertigo attack is imminent.

If your hearing is down, you are likely to be in the zone (vulnerable to having an acute Meniere's episode). Cut back immediately on all activities and take a physical rest as a preventative measure. Once you are aware of this symptom, you know you must counter the possibility of having an attack by immediately reducing stress physically, mentally or emotionally.

Tinnitus

Tinnitus is usually described as a roaring sound. You'll definitely know what sound your Tinnitus is. Tinnitus for Meniere's sufferers is created by damage to the cilia, the fine hairs in your inner ear that help with the transmission of sound to the brain. When you have an attack, the endolymph chamber is flooded with endolymph fluid, made up of sodium and potassium solution, which damage cilia hairs in the cochlea.

These little hairs send electrical impulses to the brain and once they are damaged, they don't regenerate. So unfortunately, the brain fills the void with a constant roaring sound called Tinnitus.

Once you experience Tinnitus, you can't escape it. I remember, I was on holiday in the Rocky Mountains of Colorado. It was a clear crisp blue day. The dark green fir tree branches were covered with a light dusting of snow, beneath the ground, animals sleeping in winter hibernation.

I was standing alone in deep powder snow, in natural wilderness, away from traffic, not a living soul around. My eyes could see the still quietness but the noise, for me was deafening! Tinnitus seemed to fill my inner world. I relate it to being in some industrial underworld, where the sound of roaring central air conditioning is on twenty-four hours, seven days a week, the noise ceaseless. Tinnitus is always there. You just have to accept that you will never be in a totally quiet place again.

The Benefits Of Tinnitus

The good news is, through sleep and deep relaxation, you can achieve a respite from the constant noise. I now don't feel worried about the Tinnitus as I have recruited it as a positive warning device. If I am overdoing it and it goes up in volume. An increase in Tinnitus means you body fluid has changed in some manner either by content or pressure. This means you have put your body under pressure.When Tinnitus increases in volume, think back to what you have just eaten, hidden salt, chilli, sugar, caffeine, and alcohol. Or what stress you've put yourself through lately. Take a closer look at demands and pressures of daily life. Too many late nights, worked too long on the computer, too much caffeine?

You need to be a detective, then put what ever you decide was a possible cause on your list of things to avoid. Take serious note, alter activities and take time to become acutely aware of exactly what you are doing and how you are coping. Immediately take notice and reduce whatever you're doing at the time. The attitude of using positive recruitment for all Meniere symptoms is very helpful. The more positive your focus, the less of a problem.

Tinnitus for example is a very sensitive warning signal, telling you that you are overdoing things. Or you've drunk or eaten something that is affecting you adversely. Most people don't have the benefit of Tinnitus and consequently push their bodies over the limit. Only then finding they've become chronically ill with a disease, like arterial sclerosis or heart disease.

Instead of getting depressed or down on the condition, look to use any part of it as a learning tool for a getting better and having an overall healthier life.

There are times when Tinnitus rules. That's the time to play meditation CD's to help you gain a state of relaxation. Listening to white noise CD's helps to block out and escape Tinnitus sounds. So you can do something to bring relief when Tinnitus gets too much to cope with.

Meniere's At Work

People diagnosed with an illness react in different ways. Depending on their personalities some choose to pretend it isn't happening, refusing to accept that they are ill; while others share the bad news and find comfort with family and friends. As an active, physical man, I found the diagnosis almost impossible to accept.

I saw it as a physical deterioration at forty-six. I was embarrassed to admit that I now had a weakness. So I didn't clarify my position clearly in my own business, mainly because I was confused about the full effects of Meniere's.

My suggestion is to do the opposite. Come out into the open and have some trust that there are enough good people around to support you. Tell your family. Don't hide the fact that you are having trouble with this condition. Support is exactly what you need.

Being able to be employed with Meniere's and still perform at the level you used to, can be a real problem. The fact is, there needs to be some changes. The type of job you do will determine how much change is necessary.

I know that pilots are legally not allowed to fly with Meniere's but apart from that group, you may have to negotiate your way into a position, with less demands. You will have to let your employers know how this condition is affecting you. If you are self employed, take less money and hire someone to help you.

From experience, this is the time to make significant decisions to address changes. Accept that you won't be able to function in the same way as did before Meniere's. Seek advice, from a variety of professional sources, arbitrators, counselors, lawyers, and medical specialists. Use more than one source to put your puzzle together. Then go and talk with your employer or partners. Face this issue of working with Meniere's head on and chin up.

You will need time to recover from Meniere's. Time is money. So you have to figure out how to "buy" enough time, to allow you to have a break from work. If you can't take a break from your job, then at the very least, cut back on the amount of work you are doing. Have other people step in and take over. This is the time to delegate tasks.

To share the load, to free you up. I know it is the last thing you want to do but it will only escalate to the negative if you don't. Let people know you're not feeling up to the task.

Meniere's
At Home

Having more time to yourself, is key to recovery. At home, do more for yourself and less for others in the early days. This is one time you need to think about your needs. Put 'you' first, if you can. If it's your pattern to do everything to support everyone else, you won't be able to continue doing that. If shouldering the world is your habit, then you need to learn to ask for help, and sit back a bit.

You will need time out to do activities just for yourself. A walk. A long soak in a warm bath. To move away from stress as much as you can. To do this, you need to let people around you know how you are feeling. Give them some clues. Then they can make subtle adjustments.

Doing more for yourself, is not a selfish act. When you have Meniere's, it comes down to self-preservation and finding a balance. Imagine everything in your life is compartmentalized, in equal measure. Family, work, rest, time-out, chores, holidays.

Now, at this juncture in your life, imagine giving a few of the things you usually do (and the stress that goes with then) over to someone else. You simply cannot be a doer of all things. Just thinking about this is a start.

Once you reduce your obligations to others, you can do something for yourself. Even if you do one thing for yourself in the day. The more you can do for yourself in the early stages of Meniere's, the better the prognosis is.

Time And Money Matters

Meniere's causes a definite change in financial circumstances. You will need to cut back on work. You may not be as reliable as you were. You may not be able to show up every day for work. You may have to call in sick or leave work early. When you can't predict how you will feel physically, you become less reliable in the workplace. Cutting down hours, means less in your pay packet. You will have less salary but more medical expenses, like doctor and specialist visits and pharmacy costs. In many ways, Meniere's will bring changes in your financial status, especially if you are the main earner.

If my experience helps just one of you to keep what you've worked for, this book will have been well worth the effort. A little less money and more time will give you a chance to survive financially.

If I had accepted Meniere's at that point, I would have restructured things so I could allow myself the time off work without it impacting and draining financial resources. I would not have relied on an income protection policy.

From experience, my best advice is to make significant changes to the structure of your finances in order to create a buffer for the low earning period you may find yourself in. You won't be able to bring in the same income while you are acutely sick. You may have to change jobs or quit. You may have to rely on your partner's income. You may have to borrow money. Down size the house. Cut back on expenses. Give up a few luxuries. Sell the second car. I am not kidding about this.

You need to put measures in place to protect your assets, because this is not like having flu, where you are sick for a few weeks. It is not like a heart bypass, where you need a few months. You will need at least three years working on your health, to get better. You also need to start on the road to recovery, as soon as you are diagnosed. How can you manage to spend time doing this and still look after financial obligations?

Personal circumstances are different, but there are a few basic things you can do here. My advice is to immediately look at household budgets and mortgages,then cutback and down size if you need too. Take into account accruing medical bills. Plan to restructure your present life. The change Meniere brings to a household and the time needed to recover, means you must make definite decisions early in your recovery.

You could contact management consultants to help reorganize how you operate. This is the time to use professional advisors to help you take stock of where you are going. It may not be as you dreamed, it may be better. Take your time. Use professional advisors to assist you. Face the situation and act.

Use your intuition coupled with information to ultimately determine your own future. Don't be tempted to rely on others, like income protection insurers. At the end of the day they may not be as supportive as you would expect and if you rely on them and they let you down, the effect can be financially disastrous.

The Pharmacy

The drugs prescribed for Meniere's sufferers differ from specialist to specialist and country to country. Read up and discuss your drug options with your doctor or specialist.

You will need to discuss which drugs will be best for you. Understand how specific drugs work and how they affect your body long term, it is important to find out as much as you can. Every body is different, but here's a list of the prescribed drugs I took. On diagnosis of Meniere's, my specialist prescribed Serc, (Betahistine) a blood stimulator, Kaluril (Amiloride) a diuretic, Stemetil, an anti nausea drug to help relieve the symptoms of an acute attack. He also prescribed Urea to stop the attacks as soon as they started.

Serc is the brand name for the chemical Betahistine. This drug is known to improve blood flow to the labyrinth (the bone capsule which protects and surrounds the inner ear). It is believed there may be a micro circulatory dysfunction in the inner ear due to damage done by Meniere's attacks. This means the normally independent circulatory system of the inner ear is not functioning effectively and blood flow is not efficient in the inner ear.

At the time, Betahistine was one of those controversial drugs, discussed at length as to its effectiveness for treating symptoms of Meniere's. In some trials the results indicated that not taking Betahistine was just as effective. If I forgot to take a dose, I'd experience an increase in Tinnitus and a woozy unstable feeling. Initially, these symptoms were enough for me to continue with Betahistine in the early stages. Eventually, I reduced the dosage until I no longer took any. I did this despite my doctor saying I would need to take it daily for the rest of my life. After I reduced the dosage down and came off the medication, no symptoms returned.

Again, my advice is based on my personal experience and in the realm of what drugs to take, or not, it always comes down to a personal decision. Talk with your doctor and monitor the effectiveness of drugs and be aware of possible side-effects.

Kaluri is the brand name for the chemical Amiloride. Its primary objective is to increase urinary water loss which flushes out sodium (salt).

Diuretics are documented to cause the loss of potassium in the process of flushing out the fluids. Potassium is essential for the proper functioning of the kidneys, heart, nerves and digestive system. Amiloride is often prescribed as a diuretic for long term use, as it retains potassium in the body. It's called a potassium sparing drug. So if you take diuretics on a regular basis, you need to either take a potassium sparing drug or include potassium supplements in your diet. In addition, eat a potassium rich diet as well, with such foods as garlic, onions and prunes. You can make a potassium rich broth, from vegetables like onions, garlic, carrots, and potatoes.

Diuretics, if taken for longer than six months can dramatically drop your levels of folic acid. Lack of folic acid creates a toxic amino acid associated with hardening of the arteries. So, if you suffer from high cholesterol as well, consider taking folic acid as a supplement. You can eat foods rich in folic acid. Many breakfast cereals have folic acid added.

Taking the drug Urea can be very effective for stopping attacks. Urea is a dehydrating drug. So when taken, it dramatically sucks any fluid out of the inner ear. Urea needs to be taken five minutes or so before an attack happens, in order for it to be really effective. If you are attuned to your attacks and get warning signals, like increased Tinnitus. aural fullness or a noticeable decrease in he~ Urea can stop the impending attack

When taken before important

events, Urea should enable you to participate with confidence. Urea will stop an attack happening for approximately three hours. Then when the three hours is up, one is vulnerable to an attack.

How long one would use Urea for, is debatable. You have to consider the long term effects on the kidneys. When considering this option, talk to your doctor.

Stemetil is an anti-nausea drug used in the treatment of Meniere's. This drug can minimize the impact of spinning and nausea. Stemetil can also be administered by injection.

Surgical Options

When it comes to surgical options there is not such thing as tried and true. New procedures are not necessarily break through procedures.

To chose elective surgery is a very personal decision. I didn't opt for surgery, but I know many sufferers do. The more I looked into surgery as an option, I realized that surgeons were constantly changing their views on the effectiveness of procedures. This was backed up by my specialist. I asked him about his views on the effectiveness of surgery; he said that because so much is unknown about the condition, treatments vary depending on the surgeon. This made me stop and think very carefully about surgical options.

The lymphatic sac shunt was the first operations to be offered to me. Explained as an out-patient procedure to preserve hearing and relieve vertigo. The probability of having the operation again in a year or so is high as the shunt has a tendency to become blocked and needs replacing. The shunt, as I understand, is now seen as a procedure rated by some, as having no more benefit than doing nothing at all.

Another option is Vestibular Neurectomy. After talking with a friend who had this operation for relief of his Meniere's symptoms, he said the surgery includes cutting the vestibular nerve. The vestibular nerve is the nerve of balance. By cutting the nerve any dizziness or vertigo from the Meniere's is not transmitted to the brain or to balancing receptors. This is radical surgery.

My friend was left permanently deaf in one ear and had to learn to walk again. He told me it was a shattering experience. He wasn't expecting to lose his hearing and he also wasn't prepared for the debilitating effect of having his nerve of balance cut. Having his nerve of balance cut meant he had to under go extensive long term rehabilitation to learn how to walk again.

He tells me he no longer has dizzy attacks but feels woozy and stumbles from time to time. He said, having no dizzy attacks is fine but used the old cliché: what I gained on the swings I lost on the roundabouts. For him it was not a win-win situation. The surgical option of Vestibular Neurectomy is supposed to preserve your hearing, while stopping vertigo.

Did something go wrong with my friend's operation. After surgery he had to learn how to walk again. Imagine the shock. He was supposed to retain the hearing in his right ear. Which he didn't. Talking to him, he gave me the impression that he was unaware of any possible risks or consequences of surgery. That is why all questions need to be asked before the operation. When you are prepared, you know what to expect.

I decided to stay in control and self manage. This proved to be the correct decision for me. It's a personal choice. Despite acute symptoms, don't be rushed into what may appear to be a solution at the time. If surgery is being offered to you right now, ask as many questions as you can. Look up the procedures and associated risks. Ask for a second or third opinion. There could be many successful surgical procedures to relieve Meniere's suffering. It will be interesting to see if a successful surgical procedure is universally agreed in the future, that guarantees results.

There are theories about the inner ears immune system being partly involved in Meniere's disease. The endolymphatic sac is the immune organ of the ear. This theory of immune system involvement in Meniere's, has created a trend towards surgical procedures aimed at damaging the endolymphatic sac.

The theory is, if the lymphatic sac is damaged, the immune function of the ear will be suppressed; inhibiting the immune function and consequently Meniere's attacks. On the surface, this seems logical. The latest answer is to damage the sac using a series of Gentamicin injections. Injections of Gentamicin are given through the ear drum. This procedure effectively deadens the ear. I haven't experienced the procedure, so I can't tell you what is involved in the way of discomfort. Four injections are administered in a month, effectively stopping dizziness for approximately a year. If dizziness returns, another series of injections is needed.

What Causes Meniere's Disease

There are many anecdotal reasons for the cause of Meniere's, especially from sufferers. Having an answer for why me, is a fundamental psychological building block to move forward with your life. In my case this was definitely true.

This is how I went about it. I looked into my own life and put some of my own experiences together. From a car accident to sports injury. The body retains memory or every accident or illness. Investigate your own personal history as a therapeutic exercise. To find possible causes. We need to have a sense of knowing, to help us understand possibilities. Understanding gives us personal power. So I suggest you accept your own or your specialist's evaluation and move on.

As for the cause of Meniere's, the medical professionals state that Meniere's disease has no known cause and no known origin. They are researching and investigating the possibility of causes arising from, physical trauma, as in head injuries, viral infections of the inner ear, hereditary predisposition, and allergies.

Recently, researchers have been looking at the immunologic function of the endolymphatic sac; they think immune system diseases may also be a factor. However, the underlying cause of Meniere's disease is still unknown. The research is ongoing.

Doing Life
With Meniere's
Disease

Unfortunately, Meniere's will be associated with some of the most frightening experiences of your life. The out of control nature creates such uncertainty socially, psychologically and physically. There is a lot of anxiety and fear. Any hint of an attack even for a second, still gives me a cold sweat and a racing heart! I have been there and it's terrifying.

How can 'normal' people, your doctor, your partner, your boss or friends, your insurer, understand the whirling dervish, the tumbling into hyperspace, the continual roar of jet engines in your head, vomiting, and deafness. As my doctor said, Meniere's is aggressive and confrontational. That's because it arrives without warning and it's right there inside your head.

I remember learning to sail a yacht once and the tutor told me she never had anyone seasick on her boat. Why? Because, I tell people exactly where they are going, the route they are taking and estimated time of arrival. I make a simple analogy here. What she is saying, is that, we need to know where we are going. Or we get anxious, frightened or panic. As human's we need to have a sense of direction, and knowledge of the outcomes.

With Meniere's there is the feeling of being cast adrift, with no charts or information, we move rudderless, into deep uncharted waters, our personal compass no longer registers magnetic north, and as an acute attack happens, the pointer is spinning and spinning, and we are out of control. That's the reality of Meniere's disease.

We must get back a sense of control. And we can, by being aware of our selves in relation to symptoms. From this you can create your own personal life chart and make plans with Meniere's.

Nothing changed in my condition until the moment I changed my thinking about Meniere's disease. Until the day, I decided to stand up to it and not let the disease rule my life. In short, I began to fight back using everything in my power. My will-power, my hope, my faith and trust.

I call it getting and maintaining the right attitude. First, I was determined not to end up shuffling around in slippers. I made a pact with myself that my life was not going to be relegated to pajamas and dressing gown. So, you must make an internal agreement with yourself to not give in to the condition.

So start by taking notes. Get a notebook and keep a journal. This is what I did. To gain a sense of control, I started writing everything down. I began to self-monitor and figure out what was causing the attacks. While doing my diary notes, I figured out ways to manage everything from triggers to coping methods and further, how to move forward and regain a full life without surgical intervention.

Change your mind-set. Think of yourself as an adventurer in unknown territory. You don't and won't give up on getting better. Determination is key. Do not limit yourself to feeling bad about the situation. Make a positive move towards improving aspects of your current life. Making a move in the right direction, mentally and physically makes all the difference to the outcome.

I believe I managed to counterbalance and minimize the long term effects of vestibular deterioration through physical exercise, diet, vitamins, alternative therapies and positive mental training. Creating and maintaining a personal regime is crucial. It puts you back in control. You set goals. By doing so, you are make a definite decision not to stay as you are.

By sheer creative momentum, you are

creating a counterweight to balance Meniere's and by doing so, you will move forward. That was my philosophy and it worked. In fact, you could say that I am living proof that it does work.

Create your own health regime and guarantee yourself a positive outcome. There is a lot you can do to balance your life and improve your way of life. Some call it mind over matter. Rather than accepting your situation take specific measures to improve your health. A will to get better is necessary. Rather than accepting your situation take specific measures to improve your health.

My personal philosophy on health is this: In order to affect permanent change, you have to look holistically at all aspects of your life. This is essential. You can rebalance your life with physical training, diet, as well as emotional and mental changes in attitude.

The secret is this. You can't wait until you feel better to start. You must move in a direction of health, through exercise, diet and attitude. Don't wait until you 'feel like' doing things. You have to tell your body to get going. At this point something tangible starts to happen to turn things around. You stop your body from accepting the condition as a permanent state of being. You "tell" your body, you will be healthy again. You need to adopt the attitude that, you can and will get better. Take control of your health.

Feeling down and negative suppresses the

natural ability of the body to heal itself. Don't be phased by days which are symptom heavy.

Soon, you will start to notice the attacks are less frequent, the degree of intensity is less and the gaps in between attacks is greater. The fewer attacks you have, the more normal you feel, the more hopeful you become. The more positive you feel the more energy you have. The idea is to instigate positive change on a cellular level. Your body will take note of the changes and start to respond with positive health.

I am not trying to educate medical people in the actual physiology of Meniere's disease. My Ear Nose and Throat specialist said to me, 'the cause of Meniere's is unknown and the treatments manifold, therefore straight medicine alone does not hold all the answers if indeed it holds any at all. Alternative ways of helping a long standing, ongoing, variable condition can be helpful.'

No matter how hard and difficult things are for you right now, it doesn't need to be like this forever. By making changes to your lifestyle, you can improve your health. Then Meniere's disease will not rule every moment of your life, as it may do now.

Triggers For Meniere's Attacks

Here's a hot question amongst Meniere's sufferers. What does trigger attacks? And are attacks indeed truly triggered.

Meniere's sufferers are sure attacks are triggered (caused by something specific) but there is no scientific proof to back up this hypothesis. That of course doesn't mean there aren't triggers.

When you have attacks, you want to know why they occurred. So you can stop the same thing happening again. Keep a diary to figure things out. The triggers for attacks are personal interpretations of situations and events that repeat themselves over a long time. You can work out your triggers by observing what you were doing just before an attack. Then see if this is a repeated pattern. Once you discern triggers for your attacks, avoid the situations or adapt the criteria to minimize their effects.It's that basic. As human beings, by nature, we find it very hard to accept random events especially when they are so disruptive. Rhyme and reason, we need to have it.

It is thought that anything that increases your body's blood fluid volume will in some part be responsible for increasing the volume of fluid in the endolymph. Which then eventuates in the reissner membrane rupturing, giving you an attack. This is why you should restrict anything that raises your blood pressure or changes the content of the bodies fluid.

Foods and spices that can increase your blood fluid volume are chili, curry, spices, green tea, nitrates in sausages, bacon and salami, food coloring, food additives such as monosodium glutamate, excessive sugar and salt, salted meats and fish, such as kippers, preservatives, blue vein cheeses, processed cheese, Camembert and Brie, vintage strong cheddar, processed foods, wine, caffeine, salt, sugars, spicy foods and stress are understood to affect body fluid levels.

Noise Stress

Did you know the human body never adapts to loud sudden noises or vertigo. That is why noise is so stressful and listed as a psychological stressor by psychologists. The body will adapt to most other sensory changes but never to those two. Loud constant sounds in certain cafes or restaurants can stress you out.

As you progress through Meniere's and experience more hearing loss, you will find certain environmental sounds become extremely loud. No one else hears it like this, so you have to tell your partner or friends when it's too loud for you. Shift to a quieter corner or change venues, because your hearing will not adjust to loud noise.

Physiological Stress

Physical stress on the body can cause problems. Excessive heat or cold, dehydration, overdoing physical exertion and exercise. Late nights. Dust, pollen, mould, fungus, heat, cold are triggers. Changes in barometric pressures may be a factor in having Meniere's attacks.

Excessive noise. Just plain doing too much. Lack of rest. Smoking, drinking. Emotional and mental stress. Arguments, anxiety, worry, shouldering blame, not letting go of issues, temper flare-ups, guilt, putting pressure on yourself to achieve. All and any self-defeating attitudes.

Excessive physical exercise creates physiological stress. So does any intense activity. To avoid this stress you need to limit the time for any continuous activity, to twenty minutes. Then increase this slowly, by small increments, to one hour. Put a clock on what you do. For every hour of constant activity, take a fifteen minute break. If you keep going and ignore this fact, you will enter into a zone that makes you vulnerable to attacks.

As your health improves, you won't need to monitor the time spent so rigidly. But you will always need to listen to your body.

Eye Stress

Eye stress can be a trigger for attacks. Eye muscles are connected to the vestibular system. So when your vestibular system is damaged, any excessive eye movement affects balance.

When going to the movies, check your movie and theater tickets to make sure you sit in the middle of the back rows so you can see the edges of the cinema screen or stage. Looking up suddenly can make everything spin. Look up slowly and try to control any sudden head movements. Walking down supermarket aisles is a potential problem. Have you noticed how images flickering on the edge of your vision can make you dizzy? Wearing sunglasses and walking slower will help this.

Flickering lights are a problem in stores, especially shopping malls, public foyers, galleries, airports and supermarkets. Florescent lighting, flashing, pulsing lights, neon signs, and street lights, creates both a visual and peripheral vision disturbance. You need to come up with creative solutions for light triggers. You can find ways to help cut down light intensity and disturbance created by light variants. You can wear sunglasses. Ask someone else to do the shopping. Replace flickering light tubes. Create ambient lighting using natural light and halogen bulbs.

Reduce the amount of time spent watching computer screens. I couldn't work at the computer for more than half an hour at a session. For me the computer was a trigger. If I pushed it, I'd be certain to have a Meniere's attack. I thought sunglasses could be the answer but sitting in front of a computer with sunglasses on felt weird. So I bought a screen filter to block light intensity. This helped considerably and I carefully monitored my time and increased sessions by small increments. I was able to do computer work, it just took me longer. To avoid this electronic trigger, take regular breaks when working at the computer.

Emotional Stress

Stress just doesn't exist in one form; you can have emotional, mental and physical stress. Symptoms of stress can range from tiredness to exhaustion, irritability, loss of concentration, anxiety and even sweaty palms. Don't put up with stress do something about it. Listen to your body and recognize signs of stress. Don't ignore how you are feeling.

Look very carefully at how you are reacting not just physically but emotionally in every situation. Are you emotionally overly excited or frightened, is your mind racing away, out of control. Look at everything in your life and see what is causing your stress.

Remember, emotional stress is created by the way you think, feel and react, so by its nature, it is well within your own control.

Avoiding Stress Overload

I have talked to others in the early stages of their condition and the common attitude to changing the pattern in their life is this: "I can't change anything, people rely on me. I would lose work and get behind. Then I would never get on top of it. There is no one else who can do it for me." This is the same reasoning I gave to a psychologist after she suggested I cut back on my work load. Which I didn't initially do. Meniere's forces you to change. Loading up one stress on top of another is a certain way of aggravating Meniere's. So it's better to take control and cut back on your workload.

When you're physically tired do not stack up a list of mental tasks to achieve, you must reduce the 'to do' list. Take time out.

Also if you want to reduce the amount of

Meniere's attacks you are experiencing, don't overdo one thing to the point of being exhausted. You may have a habit of being a workaholic prior to Meniere's, but you won't get away with it now. Pace yourself where you can. This is so important. Listen to your body. Be ready to back off when your body is telling you it's tired. Never work or play to a point of exhaustion. Or you can almost guarantee Meniere's will return with a vengeance.

Don't do more than one really demanding activity a day. That doesn't mean you can't do other things in the same day but make them undemanding. Try not to spend more time than you need on any one activity.

Do tasks in small time frames. For example try to limit intense conversations or meetings to approximately fifteen to thirty minutes, then move on to the next activity.

Take breaks when working on extended projects that may be taking more than an hour, then go for a small walk around the house or place of business, for a minute or two.

If you want to do something about stress, I found the following extremely helpful. The book called *Full Catastrophe Living* by Jon Kabat-Zinn, has been my mainstay during troubled times in my life. I read it cover to cover and over and over. You can use the same proven meditation techniques at home that he uses in his stress clinics.

In stressful moments, try and detach yourself from your mind, even for a minute; as though you are watching a stranger. Monitor that person (yourself) objectively. Then consider what you are doing; take positive action to minimize the stress. Change your attitude or make physical changes. Look at ALL the stressful criteria in your life and find a way of effectively alleviating it.

Seek help from a professional or read books on coping with stress. Do it and life will become very acceptable. Who knows, maybe even better than before. Meniere's is a great life teacher. Be aware, if you don't control yourself and monitor your workload and stress levels, Meniere's will take control. Meniere's is a hard task master.

Mechanics Of An Attack

You know what it's like to have severe vertigo attacks. What you may not know, is what is actually happening inside your inner ear when you are having an attack.

The main areas involved in an attack are the endolymph and perilymph compartments and Reissner membrane. Each compartment is filled with fluid which contains potassium and sodium. These two areas are separated by a membrane called the Reissner membrane.

What happens during an attack is this. The fluid volume in the endolymph cavity (potassium rich) expands and encroaches into and reduces the volume of the perilymph cavity (potassium poor); this expansion stretches the separating membrane (Reissner membrane) until it ruptures. Then the fluids of the endolymph and perilymph are mixed;

this mixture now floods the vestibular nerve (balance nerve) in the inner ear which paralyzes it. This paralysis means the signals to the brain from the paralyzed nerve in one ear are stopped or very weak. Meanwhile the unaffected healthy ear is sending out strong uninterrupted signals.

So, what you have is a strong set of signals and a weak set of signals being transmitted to the brain at the same time. This is registered in the brain as an acute vestibular imbalance. The brain then sends out signals to your body which results in acute spinning, nausea, heart rate increase, sweating and often diarrhea. This is the Meniere's attack as you know it.

Spinning Out

During the attack you would've noticed your eyes flicking back and forth. This is called nystagmus, an involuntary eye movement. This causes the spinning sensation. The nystagmus is made up of two movements, a rapid movement and a slow movement. The rapid movement is normally to the unaffected ear and a slow movement towards your affected ear. As the eye muscles are connected directly to the vestibular nerve, this imbalance of nerve signal pulsing, directly effects the movements of the eyes.

A weak pulse on one side results in a slow movement in that direction, a strong pulse from the other ear means a strong movement towards that side. So as the eyes start to flick back and forth you experience the sensation of an uncontrollable spin. These eye movements are extremely rapid. Nystagmus lasts until the affected vestibular nerve is no longer paralyzed and balanced pulses to the brain and eyes are restored. It won't and can't last forever, though at the time, the ongoing sensation feels like it will never end. But the spinning eventually gets to where the eyes are not flicking quite so badly and eventually you can keep them focused on a small dot on the wall. The settling down of the eye spinning correlates to the mending of the Reissner membrane and the recovery of the nerve of balance. The attack stops when the membrane is repaired and the normal balance of potassium and sodium are returned and the vestibular nerve is no longer bathed in the mixed fluids.

Speedy recovery of the Reissner membrane is obviously an important part of the process so anything you can do on a general health level will ensure a healthy and hopefully speedy recovery. That is why you should put measures in place to improve your health.

The whole connection between having fewer attacks, less severe symptoms, may be dependent on the overall approach to health. From rest, to vitamins and diet, to exercise. Everything you do to help yourself matters here.

There is also medical interest in certain hormones produced by the kidneys, which are by products of salt transmission. These hormones are being looked at as a possible contributing factor for Meniere's attacks. Think about what you put into your body, both as a negative and a positive. Looking after kidney function is especially important because the fluid content of the body is obviously a critical factor in the health of your inner ear. Because it directly affects the fluid volume and chemical make-up in your inner ear. In the correlation between Meniere's and kidney function, it appears that the healthier your kidney function is, the less your Meniere's symptoms are.

How To Cope During An Attack

Since that first attack and the many that were to follow, I can now suggest techniques for coping during an attack. The key to coping with attacks and reducing the effect of an acute attack, is to find ways to stop the panic and the cycle of fear. You do this effectively, by minimizing anxiety with mind control.

The mind plays a vital role in the actual attacks of Meniere's. You can minimize anxiety by being positive about the outcome of every attack. You do this throughout the attack. No matter how bad you are feeling. No matter how devastating the vertigo is. Know that the attack will pass. Tell yourself that you will be OK again. If you let the cycle of fear, anxiety and worry take you away, the Meniere's attack becomes worse.

During an attack I realized that if I allowed my mind to focus on how terrifying the ordeal was, the spinning intensified. When I controlled my mind in the attacks and didn't let it get involved in the cycle of fear, the spinning didn't seem as intensive. Detaching the mind from the experience, allows the experience to be what it is. An acute event of limited duration.

Control fear and anxiety and your attacks will appear to be of shorter duration and less intensive. Not easy, but you can do it. Look at mind control techniques. www.mindcontrol.com

Over time and after experiencing attacks, you learn to accept the fear of the possibility of an attack. When an attack happens, you use breathing techniques and mind control to carry you through. You use positive thinking to tell yourself this will pass. That you are working on your health. So soon the attack intensity will be less, the duration less and you'll have fewer attacks.

Why Meniere's Affects Hearing

Meniere's is an aggressive condition and is relentless in its destruction of your ear. So how is the hearing mechanism damaged? What happens in the ear to make it lose hearing?

Meniere hearing loss is a sensorineural nerve deafness. During an attack the cochlear hair cells of the inner ear are bathed in chemicals of sodium and potassium, due to the sudden rupturing of Reissner membrane. This rupture occurs every time you have an attack.

Unfortunately, each time you have an attack, there is permanent damage done to the hair cells responsible for transmitting sounds to the brain. These minute hair cells normally transmit sound via the hearing nerve to the hearing center located within the brain. The resulting damage to the cochlea hair cells, means the brain receives incomplete sound messages and one of the results is Tinnitus.

With each attack, more of the delicate hair cells are progressively damaged and so their ability to transmit sound is reduced and your hearing deteriorates. The longer you have Meniere's, the more hearing you lose. The intensity and range of hearing deterioration caused by Meniere's disease, is different for everyone. Nobody will experience exactly the same rate or level of deterioration.

After a Meniere's attack, your hearing should return to normal levels. As the disease progresses, your hearing will stop returning to normal levels after an attack. The hearing in the affected ear will become dramatically reduced, permanently.

Fluctuating Hearing

In the early stages of Meniere's, you will notice how your hearing fluctuates. Up one moment. Down the next. This is often accompanied by a sense of fullness in your ear, which doctors call aural fullness. This feels rather like having cotton wool packed deep inside your ear. Sound becomes muffled. Just before an attack your hearing level will drop and aural fullness will increase.

Before I was diagnosed with Meniere's

disease, I was talking on the phone to a client. He started giving me details of products. I needed to take notes, but when I swapped the phone to my other ear, I could hardly hear him. I said "Look, I've got a bad line, I can't hear you very well." I hung up and rang back on another line. When he answered, I still couldn't hear what he was saying. It was only when I swapped the phone over to the other ear, that I could hear him. What I thought was a faulty line, was a fault in my inner ear. The phone incident was the first time I noticed a real problem with my hearing.

This incident prompted me to make an appointment with an ENT specialist and the subsequent diagnosis of Meniere's disease.

While living with Meniere's, I learned to notice of any sudden change in hearing and used it as a warning sign. I figured out that if my hearing levels dropped, I was in the zone of a Meniere's attack. Also I noticed how a sudden increase in Tinnitus levels could precede a Meniere's attack. So Tinnitus and hearing levels became an internal body code I could 'read' as warning signals.

These were two important body signals I never ignored. I would act on them immediately. I'd stop what I was doing. I'd walk away from the stress. I would then go and eat, or do meditation. Have a bath. Just relax. It can take an hour or two and sometimes 3-4 days for Tinnitus levels to drop and the aural fullness to subside. Sometimes you have to be patient.

When Tinnitus levels dropped and the feeling of fullness went, I would feel 'safe' from an imminent attack. And then I would get back to normal activities. These signals became part of my management plan which I felt decreased the amount of attacks. Everything comes down to a personal choice. If you ignore these signals, you'll risk bringing on more Meniere's symptoms. If you work with symptoms and understand them as signals, then you can help yourself get better.

Sound Shock

As Meniere's progresses, the affected ear loses its dynamic range of hearing. Dynamic range is the ear's ability to cope with quick shifts in sound levels, making normal sounds seem louder than they are. This is caused by a condition called Hyperacusis; a hypersensitivity to normal sounds.

Another reason why normal sounds may be louder, is the recruitment factor associated with hearing loss. This is an abnormal perception of loudness. Have you noticed the recruitment factor in a café? You are quietly sipping decaffeinated latte and suddenly the waitress drops a handful of stainless spoons onto the tile floor.

You get a super-shock! You are experiencing the recruitment factor.

Cafes are full of spoons and china cups, so try to take a table in a quiet area, well away from extractor fans, kitchen doors and service areas. You can also try protective hearing devices such as custom made sound diffusers or ear plugs. Available from an audiologist or hearing center.

The Emotional Effect Of Hearing Loss

Interaction between people is all about how we communicate and for hearing deficit sufferers, you and me, communicating with others becomes a problem. We often miss subtle inflections or get the wrong meaning. At times, completely mishear. If there is background noise you often guess words.

Sometimes, misinterpretation can get you into some very funny conversations. At other times, it can be frustrating and detrimental to the business at hand. Hearing deficit is seen socially as a disability and by some people who refuse to understand, hearing loss is seen as a weakness. It is also associated with old age and decline of physical powers and abilities.

Deafness in the affected ear is unfortunate but it is the eventual outcome of Meniere's disease. Given the struggle that comes with hearing impairments, it's not surprising that people with hearing disabilities often become withdrawn and even aggressive. Looking closely at emotional problems associated with hearing difficulties, you may recognize some of these emotional and physiological affects in your own life: fatigue, irritability, embarrassment, tension, stress, anxiety, depression, negativism, avoidance of social activities, withdrawal from personal relationships, rejection, danger to personal safety, general health, loneliness, dissatisfaction with life and unhappiness at work. Quite a long list.

Over the years, I have experienced every one of these issues. Now that I look back at the list it is hard to accept that this is the impact it has had.

But as they all happen incrementally you do have time to adapt. There is a huge learning curve for everyone involved at home, at work and socially. Step up to the plate and be heard. Tell people to speak up or please repeat. Keep the humor going and have a laugh about it.

If you're feeling down about your hearing, I'll give you a little aside that has to do with the hearing impaired community. I went to see a film festival documentary on cochlea implants and the impact it had on the families. Before the movie started, I realized that something was very different. Normally it's quiet in the theater. Not in this one. The activity was incredible; people were smiling, waving at each other, standing up and looking around. No noise. It was a movie theater full of hearing challenged people signing to each other. This was more like a party. Two profoundly deaf friends were sitting a couple of rows in front of us. We soon caught their eye and waved discreetly. The information must have spread, that there were two hearing people in the audience. The only ones! We were the center of attention.

The documentary was insightful and I came away realizing this was a culture I knew nothing about. The hearing impaired community don't see deafness as an impairment. They see it as a difference that keeps them close together as a community. As the documentary highlighted…to hear is not necessarily an advantage.

However with Meniere's disease hearing loss can be very antisocial. At one stage, I became isolated within my own family. Even with our closely meshed love connection, my wife and two adult children did not realize, that by not including me fully in conversations or discussions; by ignoring my angst when I didn't understand some spoken words; pretending not to notice that I had misheard them. This made me withdrawn and for the first time in my life self- conscious within the family. I was being sidelined in conversations. Often they didn't bother repeating themselves, even when I asked again. Sometimes they chose not to speak loudly enough; my wife said her vocal cords felt strained from shouting at me during conversations. She had a habit of talking from inside cupboards, or from another room. They did not do this intentionally or with malice. They simply didn't understand the impact it was having on me because I did not tell them.

Isolation within the family increased daily. When they finally understood the reality of my disability and the loneliness I felt, things changed. The family gradually became more empathetic, tolerant and helpful…but I had to talk to them and help them understand how deafness affected my world. Regardless of the condition you have it's all about support and attitude. Keep your family and friends involved with your Meniere's. Don't push them away and don't give up on the social contact. Find a way around any limitations Meniere's may initially create in your life. People can be very supportive as long as you are receptive to their support.

Meniere's is a condition you can work around. Your hearing, as you know, is fluctuating and changing constantly which doesn't make you a good candidate for hearing devices. However, once hearing fluctuations decrease, you can invest in a 'hearing assist'. Miniature hearing assist devices are available in a range of customized fittings and colors. With computerization, you can attain better than normal hearing levels. So you don't have to live with a hearing disability. My virtually undetected computerized device has made a huge difference in my world. I can recommend Widex, the company I purchased the device from. Keep your family and friends involved. Keep up social contact. Find away around perceived limitations. Keep the humor level up.

The Well-Being Scale

If you think you feel bad, well the good news is you are right! The quality of life factor for Meniere's sufferers has actually been tested and quantified by research. The 'Quality of Well-Being' scale compares Meniere's disease to very ill adults with a life threatening illness such as Cancer or Aids, and that's when you're not having acute episodes.

When having acute attacks, your quality of well being is close to a non-institutionalized Alzheimer's patient, an Aids victim, or a Cancer patient…six days before death. The research quantifies that Meniere's sufferers lost 43.9% from the optimum well-being position of normal people. Meniere's sufferers are the most severely impaired non-hospitalized patients studied so far. This score reflects major impairment in mobility, physical activity, social activity and clear thinking patterns. Meniere's patients are in the significantly depressed category. This information puts experiences of depression, mobility, social difficulties and clear thinking into perspective. Maybe it's time to keep Meniere's disease in perspective. It is NOT terminal. If you have Meniere's, you get the wonderful opportunity to work on your quality of life. And to have a life. Often, people who suffer from the long term chronic condition of Meniere's, lose touch with the possibilities of their potential, restrict activities, won't try new things and become fearful of extending limits. Fear makes cowards of us all.

Adaptation is so important in moving on with life. "Go out and enjoy yourself!" Push through perceived barriers and get a larger life. I never thought I would be able to surf, learn to snow ski and snowboard, windsurf and do intensive weight training. But now I do. It is possible.

After being diagnosed with Meniere's, I was standing at one of life's crossroads. It seemed to me the decision was to wear slippers or put on running shoes. I chose all terrain walking shoes.

I had to make a definite decision to not let this disease dominate. When you don't have any guidelines, it becomes very overwhelming and challenging. You can't stand still. You learn a whole new range of physical activities that require effort, perseverance and focused balance. If you have the desire to extend yourself always look for ways around a limitation until there is no limitation. Stay focused, with purpose and always extend yourself by increments, listening to your body and don't be afraid to try.

Be prepared for setbacks. But don't give up on your goals for health and recovery. I'm not a brilliant downhill skier, but according to my old friend Al, I'm an OK snow boarder and I carve a slope like the young guys.

Make the decision. A pact with yourself. Don't let this condition dominate your life.

Cognitive Issues

Research substantiates that Cognitive ability in vestibular sufferers (Meniere's) is decreased. Here is a list of the key elements that are being researched on Cognitive disturbances in vestibular patients. Remember, vestibular covers other conditions as well, so these findings are not specifically researched for Meniere's, but for vestibular sufferers in general.

The first finding: A decreased ability to track two processes at once. Something well people take for granted. If you have two different things you want to do at the same time you will have conflicting emotions and consequent confusion. You may also find it very difficult to express this confusion. The second finding: Trouble tracking the flow of a normal conversation or the sequence of events in a story or article. The third finding: Decreased mental stamina. The fourth: Decreased memory retrieval ability. The inability to pull out information reliably from your long term memory store. The fifth: Decreased sense of internal certainty. When situations need action you have difficulty feeling confident about making a decision. Even over small issues. The sixth: Decreased ability to grasp the large whole concept. It is important to acknowledge to yourself how Meniere's has affected you. Not only in the more obvious areas of attacks, Tinnitus and loss of hearing but in the area of Cognitive capacity.

When I developed Meniere's disease, the first change I noticed in my attitude was frustration and anger over other people's demands. The people weren't the problem it was the fact of having to cope with multiple demands one after the other.

The second change, I was very tired all the time. Handling more than one job or issue at a time became increasingly hard. It was also becoming increasingly difficult to determine priorities. In a multiple demand situation, this became very obvious to me. I was even having trouble recalling details from the previous day.

I started losing that sense of rightness. You know that feeling where you are sure it's right and you can act on that sureness. I would lose the plot in an intense conversation. Talking became tiring, especially if there was more than one subject being discussed. While these changes are happening to you don't think that no one else notices. Family, friends and work colleagues will see a change. They may not know the details of how it is for you, but they will react. So this is the time to disclose your condition.

Meniere's Circles

When you have been on top of your life game Meniere's suddenly makes your life unpredictable. It's a shock to find that you can't even accomplish the smallest things, when you want to. This takes away your self-confidence. When you are trying to cope with these dynamics, you naturally practice forms of self-protection. You start living within small proven safe patterns. I call them safety circles. These circles become smaller and smaller as you become less and less confident. Over time, it becomes extremely difficult to step out side of even the smallest circle.

What you must do, if you have not done so already, is expand your social and physical parameters, little by little. Expand the dynamic of you. When you are confident look at the wider circle you have created and start expanding those new parameters. No doubt is a great motto. Have no doubt about your ability to achieve a walk around the park. Have no doubt you can have more energy if you build up your health. Or that you can achieve anything you set your mind to. When you believe in yourself, you move towards mental and physical health.

You are in a fantastic position to take advantage of what life has to offer. New skills. New Ideas. New personal power. That's why you shouldn't put your life on hold due to Meniere's.

Burning Out
Of Meniere's

After a number of years, usually four to seven, many sufferers find that vertigo symptoms subside and reduce significantly and their hearing loss stabilizing at a moderate to severe level.

This burning-out occurs in many patients. But unfortunately this is not the case for everyone. The burning-out doesn't mean Meniere's has gone; it can make an appearance at a later date. Burning-out means the hearing in the affected ear has been permanently destroyed, and the attacks are less intense or have stopped.

The risk of developing the disease in the opposite ear is estimated to be as high as thirty percent. Most doctors believe that if you are going to suffer bilateral Meniere's the symptoms usually occur in the unaffected ear within two to five years from the onset of Meniere's in the first ear. However as with most Meniere's research, these numbers are not agreed by everyone.

I must say the thought of being affected in both ears is disconcerting and I can't say it has never crossed my mind as a concern, but I don't dwell on the lottery of that probability.

My friend who had the operation, was one of the unlucky ones. He developed Meniere's in his other ear, five years after his operation. So it can happen. But the good news is, he eventually got on top of all his symptoms.

Meniere's Management

There are ways to manage your symptoms and still do the things you want to do. There is nothing standing in your way except your attitude towards your illness. Allow your spirit to rise above what may appear to be a condition with insurmountable obstacles.

Meniere's is not terminal but it's a very confrontational condition. Not terminal means you have an opportunity to live the kind of life you would like. You can decide, to persist in every way possible to obtain greater health, regardless of how uncomfortable or difficult it is at this time.

I met a man who was an outdoor survival expert. He said, in a desperate situation the greatest survival technique is to maintain a daily routine. Finding a pattern in life gives it meaning.

Meniere's creates chaos, that's why you need

to set up a daily routine. This is not an excuse to set up a comfortable pattern and live in it forever. You must set up a routine to achieve an objective, then change it to meet another objective. So you can move on towards bigger and better things.

Get Physical

Exercise yourself to wellness. The first objective I decided on was to keep physically fit. My routine was to walk twenty minutes every morning regardless of how I felt. There were times when I thought I wouldn't make it back home. At other times I felt good and so pleased to be out and going forward, rather than staying in the house.

Don't let the sensation of Tinnitus, unsteadiness and tiredness get you down. Push yourself gently and keep monitoring your response. Don't give up to fear and lethargy. It is too easy to not do anything, in order to feel safe and secure. As soon as an attack is over, get up, get on your feet, and do something. It doesn't matter how small or insignificant it is. Everything you do, matters.

Create a physical routine. During a short period of time you'll achieve the walking goal you set. Set a small goal. It can be as simple as walking down the road for ten lamp posts. Then set another goal that you are sure you can achieve easily. In time you will look back and realize you are doing things you never thought possible. Once you achieve one goal, set another. Goal setting is very important. It doesn't matter how small the goal is, as long as you achieve it. Go ahead. Keep extending physical boundaries. Setting and achieving continuous goals is the cornerstone for rebuilding your life.

The Importance Of Iron

In the beginning I decided that being physically fit was going to be the foundation for recovery. Physical confidence is one of the areas that is affected by Meniere's. You need to be physically strong and balanced. The benefit is the return of self-confidence.

I started to go to the gym regularly. I soon discovered athletes were taking serious amounts of mineral supplements. Their objective: to recover quickly from exhaustive body work outs, build body mass and stamina. This constant process of building strength meant they understood how to effect change in their bodies. This principle interested me as I wanted to rebuild a healthy body. I decided to emulate their exercise plans, vitamin and diet regimes, to see what it could do for Meniere Man.

I started with light weights and over time, I added small weight increments to my routine. After six months my balance and strength had increased considerably. Working your muscles to the point of muscle exhaustion is the objective. Work to failure and be congratulated for a job well done. Rest for thirty seconds and begin again. It is really fascinating to feel your body recover in thirty seconds. It showed me how quick the body recovers. I started to look seriously at my nutrition, not just to avoid salt, but to replenish my body, so it would be well equipped for regeneration after attacks.

Research on weight bearing exercise in retirement homes, shows that immediate benefits are obtained with light weight - bearing exercise. In a very short time, elderly who exercise with weights, get stronger and more independent. They don't fall over as much and they are far more active. The benefits of weight bearing exercise are too many to ignore. And there is no age, sex or level of illness that should stop you getting the benefits by doing regular weight-bearing exercise. Weight training improves blood pressure, muscular strength, bone density and your nervous system. Plus the psychological benefit of personal confidence and self esteem. Weight training creates an asymmetrically balanced body. This helps the body counter and compensate for any unsteadiness.

Don't be put of by the word gym. Make the effort to go outside the home to do your exercise. You go to the gym to workout. To work on individual muscle groups with real intensity. This makes the work outs far more interesting. The aim is not to become huge and muscle bound, but to focus intently on what you are doing.

This intense focus made me realize how much my mind affects my ability to achieve goals. A negative thought, while lifting at your maximum, meant failure in the lift. A positive thought, with the same weight meant a successful lift. The mind experience of failure and success repeated over and over again was so obvious; you just couldn't ignore its principle. Think positively. Haven't we all heard that before. However the experience of failing and succeeding physically made the principle of positive thinking all the more potent.

I did improve my strength by three times; my body was equally strong on both sides. And I was windsurfing and skiing. So, not too bad for a Meniere's guy who thought that a twenty minute walk, nine months prior to that, was beyond him.

The important factor is having a measurable and quantifiable means of seeing progress, where you're in control and making a considerable difference to your quality of life. The intense focus on weight bearing exercises keeps you in the present, in the now. True intense concentration in the present creates a state where you no longer hear your Tinnitus and for moments of time you don't register the symptoms.

Building strength for body balance, taking the right health vitamins and watching your diet are the right steps to positive health. Think of yourself as getting healthier and more positive with Meniere's.

My gym training wasn't all success though! I made errors of judgment. There were times when I did too much exercise and had more Meniere's attacks. Learn to pay attention to the signals your body gives you. Take a rest. Sit down for fifteen minutes and let your body recover. Respect what your body tells you.

Balance Training

My next trainer had an interest in physical rehabilitation. He followed a style of training created by a man called Paul Chek. An American trainer who was responsible for looking after the top grid iron athletes in the USA. The gridiron teams would send injured players to Paul Chek with the knowledge that he would have them back out on the field, faster and fitter than any one else in the rehab business.

He created a rehabilitation system based on core balance training. He believed that the key to physical performance was based in strengthening the human core. This core training is now very popular and well recognized as essential for optimal bio-mechanics. You can find these same principles in other exercise programs such as Pilates. Most gyms have core training programs.

If your body is not strong in its core muscle function your imbalance will be more pronounced. As you know your vestibular system is affected by Meniere's so you need to ensure your body balance receptors are strongly developed. Correct body posture and specific identification with your body's infrastructure will help compensate your imbalance issues. Bad body posture for example, will be telling your brain you are imbalanced. To give your body good balance you need isometric training to improve your body posture. Trainers can show you how to do specific exercises to achieve this.

If you combine isometric training with core muscle training, you will be able to achieve body balance. To a very high degree. Even to the point of being able to stand perfectly still on the top of a large round exercise ball. And it is possible to do. The benefits of training will show up in every cell of your body. Regardless of age or sex.

All knowledge gained by trainers will assist you well after you leave the gym. I still use the information in simple physical activities. How to pick things up off the floor properly by bending your knees and contracting your stomach muscles to support the back. Once you've been shown how to stand evenly and in balance, protecting and strengthening your back is something you'll continue to do quite naturally.

With your body balanced and strong, every cell of your body, including the inner ear, will benefit. A healthy fit body has the ability to heal more quickly. Physical training enables your body to recover its balance faster after attacks. You will really start to feel the difference in your health.

If you liked sports, or exercise before you were diagnosed with Meniere's, don't stop. The importance of stimulating the sensory body through physical activity will help you improve your balance and recovery. Medical researchers are finding that intense exercise within the first six months of an injury or onset of a condition, gives patients a greater expectation to recover physical losses.

In the beginning I was having trouble bending over and picking up a ball and throwing it to my daughter, without feeling dizzy. Then one year later, after exercising in the form I have described, I was going wind surfing with her regularly. Without core balance training, I would never have gone out on the water in strong winds to give it a go.

I have gained so many benefits from a progressive controlled weight training program that I urge you to look into it as soon as you can. Don't wait until you feel better to start. As long as you have patience with yourself, understand that you won't feel great to begin with. You may feel dizzy during a workout, or have a vertigo attack after. Chances are, you would feel the same whether you were working out or lying in front of the T.V. So resist the urge to blame physical activity if you feel unwell that day.

Work with a nutritionist and a weight program designed for you. Don't forget to inform them of your condition. A gym will design a specific program for you. Ask about a core balance program. In some gyms individually tailored fitness plans are free with membership.

The first four months of any gym membership is where the likelihood of dropping out happens. Your muscles get sore and it can be hard to find the motivation to go. That is why a personal trainer is good. If you can afford one. Many gyms offer free consultations with personal trainers who help you set a program when you sign up. Whether your trainer is there at every session, or available to monitor your progress, you will benefit from their expertise and discipline. Often they become great personal friends. They care about what you are doing and how you are. They offer inspiration and motivation. Knowing your trainer is at the gym waiting for you, means you're less likely to cancel out. Trainers help you get results. You'll not only feel better. You'll look younger, fitter and stronger too.

Vitamin Power

I heard a doctor talking on a radio talk back program and it made sense. He said, that every illness and condition is caused by a lack of minerals and/or vitamins in the body. Since we can't get all these from foods, he recommended vitamin and mineral supplements.

The gist of what he said made sense to me. I started reading up on vitamins and their properties. I paid special attention to the chemical make-up of each vitamin and its role in the body. The more you understand the importance of how specific minerals and vitamins effect your well-being, the more you'll be able to help yourself to obtain maximum health.

I found out that stress depletes the adrenal glands. So I started taking vitamins to support the adrenal glands. I was determined to step up my physical goals and improve my health.

To trial the effect of additional vitamins I

chose the most common ailment. The common cold, a sure sign of a weak immune system. I decided to see whether I could work out a vitamin regime that would give me an obvious result. No more colds or flu would be my goal.

I decided to support my immune system by taking high levels of Vitamin C and Vitamin E. I started taking 1000cc of Vitamin C a day and over a month increased it to 4000cc a day. As an antioxidant I took 24 mg of Vitamin E. The end effect was a great immunity to colds.

I was very encouraged with this and looked further into what else I could do to help myself with Meniere's disease. Complex vitamin B assists with nerve regeneration, reducing stress, depression and picking up energy levels. Essential Fatty Acids reduce inflammation and assist with nerve transmission and manufacture and repair of cell membranes. Essential Fatty Acids come from fatty fish like salmon and vegetable oils. As well as eating a diet rich in oily fish, I took fish oil and flax-seed oil in a supplement form three times a day. Also, a multi-vitamin once a day. In time my vitamin drawer was often a source of humor for my friends, because of the volume of vitamins I consumed.

My daily vitamins regime included the following supplements. **Vitamin B Complex:** assists the nervous system to reduce stress, depression and picks up energy levels. Supports the immune system. **Vitamin E:** Promotes healing; 24 mg spread through out the day at meals. **Essential Fatty Acids:** regenerates cell membranes, reduce inflammation and assist in nerve cell transmission. Fish oil liquid or capsules 1000 mg 3 times a day. Flax seed oil 5 mls 3 times a day. (Use as a dressing for salads, but do not heat the oil and cook with it!) **Vitamin C:** supports the kidneys, liver and immune system. 2-4000 cc spread throughout the day and at least one hour before or after food. I take up to 4000 cc a day if I am feeling like I am getting a cold, but normally I take 2-4000 cc a day regularly to keep my immune system supported. **Multi-vitamin:** One a day. My choices are Swisse Men/ Women Ultivite, or TwinLab. These brands have documented high quality sources. I know this level of vitamins works. My daughter caught flu and was bed ridden for five days, then my son, then my wife. I had Meniere's but no flu and this pattern was repeated often during winter. I can only recall getting a mild cold and flu once in the last six years.

Additional Supplements

If you are going through a particularly stressful time, take vitamins to specifically support your adrenal glands and immune system. Calcium, zinc, niacin, oil of primrose, borage oil, selenium, magnesium, carnitine, chromium, co-enzyme Q10. And extra B6, B12.

Another thing. Don't forget to drink plenty of mineral water everyday. Not tap water! Pure, uncarbonated (carbonated has higher salt content) mineral water. Read the label and go for lowest salt, highest magnesium. Evian water has a high content of magnesium.

Eat. Drink. Play.

You are what you eat. And drink! What you put into your body, the vitamins, minerals, water, matters to your Meniere's health. Here's why.

The inner ear when healthy, has its own independent regulatory fluid system and is not affected by any chemical or blood fluid volume dynamics of the body's fluid system.

Meniere's results in the loss of the inner ears independent fluid function. The damage from attacks means the inner ears fluid system is no longer independent from the rest of the body. This results in the inner ear's fluid volume and chemical concentration being subject to the chemical make up of the body's blood fluid. Any fluctuation of the body's blood/fluid volume and chemical makeup can cause symptoms in the ear, such as the sensation of fullness, pressure and Tinnitus. It can also give you dizziness and imbalance. This does not mean an attack is eminent, these are extra symptoms that you will experience.

Eating is one of life's great pleasures and you can keep enjoying food. However you won't be able to indulge in salty foods because salt is one of the main elements linked to vertigo attacks. So lets look at why salt is the bad boy in food.

The inner ear is bathed in a very specific concentration of sodium and potassium. And if you change this delicate balance, by eating food high in salt (sodium) which in turn is absorbed into your blood stream, you are setting yourself up for a fast delivery of a high concentrated sodium solution into the defenceless inner ear.

This results in an imbalance of sodium and potassium concentration. The inner ear desperately tries to even out these concentration levels by diluting, with water, the chamber, with the highest concentration of sodium. This, in turn, expands one of the compartments. As a result, the separating Reissner's membrane becomes so extended, that it ruptures and you have a Meniere's attack.

This is why you must limit salt intake to around 1000 mg or less a day. This level of salt represents a low salt diet. Some salt is vital for body function. So you don't want to have a zero salt diet. You just need to control the intake to around 1000 mg a day.

Get to know how much salt is in raw and

processed foods. How much salt you ingest in a day needs to be monitored by you. There are no salt police about! Restrict your daily salt intake or suffer the consequences.

I heard one of the top vestibular specialists say that he recommends that his Meniere's patients don't eat out at restaurants because they cannot control the amount of salt in the food. I disagree with this. You need to get out and enjoy life like everyone else does. Don't stop eating out for fear of eating the wrong thing and aggravating Meniere's. Don't stop participating in social occasions. It is imperative to keep up social contact and not fall into a reclusive style of living.

Restaurant food is about choice. Look at your favorite restaurant menus and make your own dietary decisions, based on the salt content of the dish. Here's my advice on eating out.

Italian Food: Look for meals that don't have sauces on them. Try the fish or veal without sauces or ask for sauces on the side.

Fast Food: All fast foods are out. They all have way to much salt added to the crumbs, batters, sauces and dressings.

Japanese: A terrific way of eating. The sashimi, nigiri and tempura are good sources of food with low salt. Salads are also good. Don't eat the shabu-shabu as the stock base is salted. Miso soup is heavy in added salt. Stay away from seaweed soups and sauces. Wasabi (hot green horseradish paste) in the sushi is my only vice and I suffer from increased Tinnitus as a result.

Japanese is my food of choice. There is low-salt soy by the way. Some establishments have it. Check it out, or ask for it. Sushi without soy sauce takes a little getting used to. Instead of using soy you can dip food in mirin, a fermented rice wine which tastes delicious,

Alcohol: Minimize beer and wine to a glass. I have found that spirits are out, as spirits and liqueurs seem to increase Tinnitus and my hearing drops significantly. I suspect it is due to the fact that the high alcohol content raises your blood pressure, which will affect your inner ear system.

French Cuisine: Sauces feature heavily in French regional dishes. Choose simple dishes without sauces. Salt is a major taste ingredient for sauces in particular. Even butter contains salt.

Korean: The dishes cooked in the restaurant kitchen are full of spices and salt. But if you order food and cook it yourself at the table, in the traditional manner, you are in control. All the meat, vegetables, and spices come on separate plates. It's a fun way to eat with friends and you are in control. Forget the spices and you'll be OK. Again don't go for anything that has sauces or has been pre cooked.

Chinese It's often loaded with msg (mono sodium glutamate) and table salt. Steamed Dim Sums are great if they don't contain msg or salt.

Try a few different restaurants to find the places that don't use msg or heavy salt.

Indian food Now this is unfortunate as I can't think of an Indian dish that does not have a sauce containing salt. I now only eat Indian curries at home. I make them myself, no salt and a limited amount of mild or medium strength curry powder. Don't use curry paste as this is often very high in salt. You can make an excellent curry without salt by using limes, ginger, lemon grass, garlic, shallots, tumeric, cumin and pepper.

Cafes If you're an urban person this is a stimulating environment, but if you're a Meniere's sufferer, drinking coffee can be an issue. But, you can have your cake and coffee too. If you drink decaffeinated coffee, you can enjoy the social benefits of cafe life without issues.

Your overall health will be greater and your Meniere's symptoms less, if you apply a few simple rules of healthy living. Limit alcohol. Have a low salt diet. Eat more complex carbohydrates which provide slow burning energy for your body.

Sugars in processed foods cause sudden sugar spikes and lows that you want to avoid. With Meniere's you are more sugar sensitive than normal. You will notice that sugar affects your body in a negative way. I found that even a teaspoon of simple sugar added to my coffee or sprinkled on cereal, affected my hearing immediately and caused an increase in Tinnitus .

Cut out simple sugars, (like soft drinks, candy, sweets, jams and cakes) as they are absorbed into your blood stream quickly. This is really important. Eat complex carbohydrates rather than refined sugars.

Take note of hidden sugars. Packaged goods have the sugar content per serving. Note also, that some low fat foods contain more sugar to add taste. So get into a habit of reading the labels on products and comparing brands.

Think of having a low salt and low sugar diet, not in terms of restrictions, but rather for optimal health. Less salt means less issues with blood pressure and hypertension. Less risk of a stroke. Low sugar means less risk of coronary disease and diabetes and better weight management. Less sugar and salt means you reduce your risk for most major health issues.

In the early stages of Meniere's disease, I cut down on spicy foods. I was made aware of my body's reaction to foods and additives through increased Tinnitus levels. Hot spices increase the blood volume in your body, which affects the fluid pressure in your inner ear. Cutting out spicy foods is not a permanent measure. Later you will be able to eat a bowl of chillies! But while in the acute stages of the disease, when you are prone to vertigo attacks, I would leave those out. Replace for taste: Herbs for spices. Your meals don't need to be bland and tasteless. There is a garden of herbs to give food a piquant taste, like parsley, basil, coriander, mint, chervil, tarragon, marjoram.

Look for foods that are primary products such as vegetables, whole grains, and fresh protein. Try to cut out or limit down foods that come in a tin or packet. Avoid ready cooked or processed foods like spaghetti sauce in a jar or dried soup in packet. Read the labels and choose the lowest sodium content.

Meals should consist of a protein, complex carbohydrates with no wasted calories from refined sugars and processed foods. Fresh vegetables, fish, chicken, meat, fruit and grain cereals and breads are smart choices.

Another huge factor in promoting health, is giving up smoking. You can't afford to light up, because smoking restricts blood vessels. This affects the ability of blood to circulate efficiently in the inner ear. Limiting blood supply to anywhere in your body is a problem. Your ear needs the healing substances which are carried in your blood. If your ear doesn't get what it needs, it's in a vulnerable state and more likely to be prone to ongoing Meniere's trouble. Make sure your body gets as much healthy blood as possible. Your body is constantly replacing itself, so make sure you take the opportunity to rebuild yourself stronger and better than ever before. If you are a smoker and have Meniere's disease, stop smoking.

Maintain your blood sugar levels by making sure you eat a balanced breakfast of protein and complex carbohydrates. Don't skip meals during the day or leave long gaps without eating. Think in terms of six small meals instead of the traditional three meals a day. This keeps your blood sugar levels up. Eating a big meal will spike your blood sugar levels, causing feelings of tiredness, lethargy and even depression. So remember to keep your body fuelled up with the right stuff.

Environmental Equations

While figuring out the management of Meniere's, I went back to nature. I found water especially therapeutic. Relaxing in the bath. Standing under a shower. Swimming in the ocean, or sitting near a lake or a river. The benefits of mountain and sea are universally acknowledged through civilizations as places of rejuvenation.

Rather like the old methods of cures, where the sick were ordered to take rest in the mountains or by the sea, I also discovered the benefits of mountain air at high altitude. How taking family time together, away from the city, the air crisp and skies blue, rejuvenated body and soul.

I wondered why getting away from the city, made me feel so much better. Scientific research demonstrates that the content of ion in the air is of great importance to air quality. People living in forests, near waterfalls and the seashore enjoy much better quality air and freshness because the Ion content in these places is 1000 times more than office buildings and urban residential areas.

The oxygen combined with Ion is active and easily absorbed by human organs, which benefits the body and revives the spirit. In relation to human health, they say forest, waterfall has a content of 100,000 -500,000 Ion S/CC per milliliter, aiding spontaneous recovery. Mountain and seashore have 50.000-100,000 Ion S/CC and fields 5,000-50,000, enhancing immunity. As compared with enclosed urban and residential areas 40-50 Ion S/CC which are known to induce psychological disorders, headaches and insomnia.

Does a negative environment, polluted and crowded cities defer reaching our optimum sense of well-being and delay our healing? It may do.

With health in mind, if you can't get to the mountains or sea occasionally, take a long shower, take a walk on wet, dewy morning grass. Stand in a warm shower of summer rain. Sleep in a well-ventilated room. Consider purchasing a remote controller air cooler/humidifier with an ionizing feature to create your own healthier environment.

Alternative Therapies

In the process of getting better, I formulated a vitamin regime, a fitness plan and changed my diet. I had come along way in my personal self-management program but I was still a little frustrated by not being able to do more than one intense activity a day. I was pleased with the progress in training and my health so far. But I still wanted to be able to do more to try to reduce down the vertigo attacks and eventually be symptom free. To overcome this disease. That was my ultimate goal.

Acupuncture

The personal trainer I was working with went to an acupuncturist whom he highly recommended. A Chinese doctor, now in his sixties, who had once been a child athlete chosen for the Chinese international acrobatic team. He trained and performed around the world from five years of age until he was twenty one. He later went to the medical school in Shanghai. And eventually swam to Hong Kong and then later immigrated to Australia. He sounded like an interesting person to meet at the very least. So I did.

I always remember this. The old linoleum covered floor of the corridor led to a glass paneled door. As I entered a bell rang. The front room of his office was stocked with Chinese medicinal herbs in glass cabinets. Large glass jars sat on the counter full of herbs and fungi. A laminated acupuncturist's chart hung on the wall. Energy flow lines were illustrated running around the body like electrical wiring, little red, black and yellow dots indicating electrical junction points, areas for precise needle work. Acupuncture is an ancient Chinese practice for tuning the body's energy fields and is widely recognized in the west as a legitimate form of medicine.

The acupuncturist was a very enthusiastic and skilled acupuncturist and as I got to know him better, he showed me his acrobatic manoeuvres, learned as a child in China. One of them was a handstand on a rotating, rolling office chair. He stayed that way for about five minutes. Talking to me about China with his hands gripped around the armrests of his chair and suspended upside down. perfectly still, except for the trousers that slid down from his ankles exposing his white socks and black shoes. As he came down he said " I'll always be able to do that, doesn't matter how old."

I began to trust this man and we went into the more advanced stages of acupuncture. "You are able to do this."He told me I was able to with stand pain and would benefit from having some more."I have looked up your Meniere's in my journals. This Moxibustion would be very beneficial for you. It will help this Meniere's." So my initiation into the Chinese healing art of Moxibustion began.

"Sit very still,when the pain gets to six out of ten let me know, if you can get to eight or nine that would be even better. I'll just cut your hair a little bit here at the top of your head." Then he put something on top of my head and lit it. I sat very still. Soon I smelt incense, not perfumed incense, but a medicinal herb smell.

I waited. Nothing. No pain. Then, a little tingling on the top of my head. Then came pain. I counted the pain as a four. Where was he? He had this ability to disappear for long periods of time. The pain was in my skull bone. When he extinguished the moxi fire the pain slowly lifted. He said, Moxibustion is very good. I burn special Chinese herb on your head. He laughed.

A few days later, I was at home, looking at

the top of my head with a mirror. I had a scab the size of a twenty cent coin, three centimeters across. I felt it and it moved a little. The scab came off and I couldn't believe it. I had a hole in my head shaped like China. It looked as if a this area of my scalp had been burnt down to the bone. I didn't go back for further moxi treatment!

Despite the scar on my scalp, I felt so much better from all the treatment. The acupuncture sessions were a turning point for me. Even after I had stopped the sessions, I still had positive benefits from acupuncture. My attacks became less frequent and far less distressing. The acupuncture treatment raised my energy levels up and my skin color and tone were healthier looking. I looked and felt much better.

I do believe the acupuncturist cared about my health and was doing his utmost to help me. But the moxi hole in the head and the promise of curing my baldness took it out of the realms of believability. I have read since that the head is the one place where a practitioner should not burn moxi cones. If you choose to go this route, a registered acupuncturist will advise you on treatment methods and options.

Hypnotherapy

Hypnotherapy was my next adventure into Meniere relief. I was recommended to a therapist, who unlocked childhood traumas. These forgotten child dramas apparently create major problems in your adult life. Releasing these blocks through therapy could greatly assist adult healing. Well this was what I was told.

I was on the healing journey, so along I went. I thought maybe my childhood was dramatic enough to have caused some blockages. Maybe I've been blocked since childhood and now in later life Meniere's is the result. I had no idea, but neither do the best medical researchers in the world.

I found myself counting backwards, then recounting events from childhood. The first question I had to think about was how did I feel when I killed a chicken with my slug gun? I was surprised it died with its feet in the air. I was just shooting with my gun. I didn't think death was part of the game. He stared at me.

I resisted tears for three sessions and left a little wiser but not a little cured. I must still be blocked but I'm alright with that. I didn't complete all the sessions because, to be honest, I wanted to feel a difference. Hypnotherapy didn't make any difference for me. But as the saying goes, different strokes for different folks.

Cranial Manipulation

There is a gentle art of cranial manipulation. I asked around and found a man who was almost impossible to get an appointment with. He was getting good results with all sorts of patients. A month later my appointment time arrived. I was full of expectation and hope. I walked into his office, but he was a she, as he had gone on sabbatical. I lay down and she applied very light and sensitive pressure on my head, using the palms of her hands. In this way she 'read' my skull. She accurately identified an old but significant trauma to my skull that I had happened to me. She said it was probably a major accident as the impact must have been severe. That my neck was currently out of alignment and had been for a long time.

I was impressed with the diagnosis and subtle manipulation. I left an hour later. I went back three times but I didn't notice any real change to my condition. I never went back for a fourth. Some people persevere with cranial manipulation and claim noticeable results.

Massage

If you decide on having a course of massage therapy, it's important, to only have gentle massages. Deep tissue sports massage can be stressful on a physical level. The key to preventing issues, is to stipulate what you don't want. You don't want neck manipulation of any description. Gentle massage is great though, as you will find that your shoulders, back and neck muscles will be tense from the continual automatic adjustments your body is making for balance.

I went for regular full body massage sessions with great results. Any imbalance in my muscles were making got corrected. I slept better. I was less tired. I had an overall sense of well-being.

My masseur was a young man who had literally fought his way back from the dead. I heard his intriguing personal story over many massages. His story was of a motorbike accident in his mid teens. This traumatic event left him in a coma for two months. He was expected to have extensive brain damage as his skull was severely crushed. When he woke up he had a large metal plate in his skull. Then, rehabilitation and after two months sent home to be a living but mobile vegetable. He refused to accept his physical and social restrictions. So six months later, he booked a flight overseas, paying for tickets with some of his accident compensation money. His plan was to survive on his own, away from the restrictive prognosis his doctors and family had.

Two years later, he arrived back home having traveled the world, living on his instincts and very little money. He most definitely was not a vegetable as doctors had predicted. He had gained a black belt in a combat martial art. And now, here he was. Five years after his accident, living with a beautiful girl in his own house. He was massaging for a living while studying to be an osteopath. Despite the odds stacked against him, he was living a spectacular life.

His complete dedication and belief in his own ability to affect recovery, was a poignant lesson for me. And he was very entertaining with a great sense of humor. It is fascinating how many inspirational stories come from everyday people overcoming incredible obstacles. One day, while I was having a massage and talking through the hole in the table, his little pet rabbit hopped under the massage table. I was looking down as this rabbit was looking up. A white rabbit staring at me with those clear red eyes like glass marbles, that only rabbits have.

"What made you get a rabbit for a pet?" I asked."Well I do kids magic shows in the weekends. I am a clown and I do magic tricks with the rabbit. But I've stopped doing it because I don't like children. Way too noisy and active!"

He went on to say that to conquer his fear of timidity, he took up flame blowing. "You mean where you take a flammable liquid in your mouth and light it as you blow out?" I asked. "Yeah that's the one. Someone at the last party put the wrong propellant in the container and it burnt too soon, so I burnt my face and arm." I thought his face looked a little red but hadn't thought that much about it. "Only did it three weeks ago." His burns had almost healed. "I visualized my face and arm healing, every two hours", he said. Later, when I turned over and had a close look at him, it was remarkable. He showed me a photo of the burns soon after he had been burnt. The recovery was amazing considering the small time frame. The masseur had told me his secret for recovery. To overcome obstacles, you must believe in the power of positive visualization. He also believes in creating his own reality and constantly extending himself. So do I.

Biofeedback

When I was first diagnosed, a psychologist recommended a few sessions of biofeedback monitoring. It helps you train the parts of your body that you have control over. For example, your thoughts, your ability to relax you muscles.

Sitting in a chair, I was connected to a small machine by electrodes. I could not feel any pain or sensations during this monitoring. I was asked to close my eyes and visualize the figure 1: breathing in to the count of three and out to the count of three. Thirty minutes later, the psychologist explained to me what levels of relaxation I had obtained and the length of time I was the most deeply relaxed.

Over a six week period, I soon became familiar with different levels of relaxation. This method of monitored meditation, enabled me to quantify the depth and length of relaxation.

At home, I practiced the same meditation method for total relaxation. Practicing with biofeedback made me aware of relaxation levels. I took every opportunity to relax. Waiting at the doctors, sitting in the park, waiting for a friend.

Before I experienced biofeedback, I thought that sleeping was the only time my body was rejuvenated. Now I know I can revive my energy levels through deep relaxation. I found it very beneficial as a tool for de-stressing.

Meditation

Stress is a major factor in Meniere's and in modern life. I have found meditation an essential tool for coping with both stress and Meniere's.

Meditation is great but you must practice regularly. As soon as I felt I was improving, I'd get busier and forget to do meditation. This is common. As soon as you start to feel better, you tend to forget about what made you better. So you re-instate the meditation disciplines again. Human nature I suppose. But the idea is to make meditation an integral part of your daily habit. You need a method of meditation practice that you can do everyday, without going to an ashram or hall.

I was keen to find some method that I could do conveniently and privately at home. Then by happenstance, I was having my skin looked at microscopically by my skin specialist. I was talking to him about the relaxation method called biofeedback and asked whether he had heard of it."Yes." A man of few words, but a keen eye. He told me he had another form of meditation that he had been practicing regularly for a couple of years.

He gave me a tape to listen to. The meditation program was made up of a series of tapes which you progressed through over weeks months and then years. The starter set sounded like ocean waves rolling onto the sand; while a deep sounding voice-over guided you through the meditation.

During the meditation sessions my Tinnitus was completely masked. The tapes gave me a strict time period that was just for meditation; the tapes were half an hour per side. A total of one hour a session. So I could easily plan the session into my day. After spending an hour meditating I was alert and my energy levels restored. I would feel refreshed and ready to do things. The benefits I received from meditation were, less stress, less Tinnitus, positive life perspective, increased energy levels, a sense of hopefulness, and a greater sense of oneness with life. All this and the luxury of having a quiet time to myself, Meditation became a breeze. I could put on a tape everyday at whatever hour I chose and all the family left me on my own. I was totally blissed out. Meditation became a sanctuary I escaped to everyday. The relief of not focusing on Meniere's is a gift worth giving yourself.

Having the tapes was a great way of staying at home and meditating without having to put any effort out. An hour a day of meditation will put your life into perspective, guaranteed.

At the time of writing, I am re-reading a book called *Full Catastrophe Living* by Jon Kabat-Zinn. It's a book about how to cope with stress, pain and illness using mindful meditation. Jon is a Professor of Medicine emeritus at the University of Massachusetts Medical School. His book is straight forward, and practical. I used his meditation CDs' on a daily basis.

A Strategy For Wellness

There comes a time when you must break out of your old habits. Early on in my personal history of Meniere's, I caught myself rushing around the car to put petrol in the tank as though it was an emergency. The only thing waiting for me on the other side of the car was a petrol cap. Getting into the car and putting the key in the ignition was all done in the most efficient manner. My whole being was a study in time efficiency. And it didn't stop in the gas station it happened at home.

I wondered why I was so rushed. Then it occurred to me. I did everything in a hurry. There was no differentiation between any activities. Talking with a colleague or friend, I was always impatient, I wanted to finish the conversation as soon as possible. I was wired. It was my life. I powered on. I thought it was still exhilarating.

It wasn't until sometime later, that I realized this physical stress was physically contributing to my attacks. This meant if I wanted to limit my attacks, I had to change these old patterns. This made me stop and look at everything I did in order to identify what was contributing to my stress. The gas station rush was just one of the revelations in my daily activities.

So, become aware of yourself; look at things you are doing in your life, you may have habits and patterns you got away with before, but now you have Meniere's, they will be your stress factors.

Look at how you drive your car, eat your food, and talk to friends and family. Do you take your time or is it all in a rush and never ending. Only you know and you have to adopt a new strategy of personal awareness. You'll need to do a mental and emotional re-evaluation. You need to re-invent your own personal operating manual for day to day relations with friends, family, business colleagues and yourself.

If you need professional stress management help, then get it. You may chose to work with a psychologist to help you change patterns of thinking and behaviors. This is key to personal control. Adapt and be conscious of what you are doing to create stress in your life. Lessen stress every minute of every moment. By reducing stress, you will find your Meniere's attacks will lessen in intensity and duration.

However, as I discovered, making changes means everyone around you will be affected. In relationships we get used to automatic responses from people in certain situations and learn to rely on those responses. Changing patterns initially can be stressful in itself, but necessary, if you are going to get your life back.

When I realized what a big impact stress had on Meniere's symptoms, I made definite changes to lessen the stress and as a consequence I became unpredictable in my personal and business relationships. I no longer expressed extreme dissatisfaction or got involved in conflict. No more rushing to complete tasks. Some tasks I left uncompleted and never finished. I stopped projecting linear time frames and participating in multiple tasking. You can imagine how unsatisfactory this was in business and in personal relationships. I could no longer be relied on to complete tasks. This was only the start of my restructuring. Some of it extreme and inappropriate but it was a revolution for me and when you have a revolution it can go a bit too far one way.

I tried to reach a balance on the types of responsibilities and tasks I could and couldn't achieve. Ultimately one needs to address just how, why and what you are doing on a daily basis. And of course, how your actions affect others.

Talk To Yourself

The first and most important thing you can do right now, is this. Start this minute to develop an new attitude and a belief system that will allow you to overcome physical, emotional and mental barriers. It is vital you begin to reprogram your mind into a healthy state of being. Move forward to a positive future. Just to get you started, you may like to try my mantra.

I am not my disease.
I feel good about who I am.
I am healthy.

I repeat these lines everyday aloud, three times a day, for about five minutes. Each time I say a line, I visualize a positive image of myself.

You need to believe in each phrase as you repeat it. You can use this mantras or create your own. Keep it short so it's easy to remember.

Mantras really help. In the beginning I felt completely invaded and controlled by Meniere's and it was a real struggle to retain my identity. After doing the mantra, I began slowly to feel more positive about myself and my situation.

It is important to begin as soon as possible. Make this your first step to believing, not only in yourself, but in believing that you will not always feel this bad. Soon you'll feel in control of your life again.

The Hi Friend

When you realign your personal energy and attitudes, you may come to understand a new term in the social order...the Hi Friend. The person who you decide to not give out time and energy to as you previously did. The Hi Friend is just someone you say hullo in passing to. They don't expect all the effort you think you need to give out. In fact the simplicity of defining time is how you save time. And who you give time to.

You come to prioritize, because you no longer give your personal time and energy endlessly. You can't afford to. It's called personal conservation. When you practice conserving, you are not limiting yourself. You are just being more selective in personal output. And you become less stressed. We realize we don't have to do as much for people as we think. You don't have to make everyone like you. You don't have to do so much for people at the expense of yourself.

You'll realize by cutting back on giving out

your time, energy and effort to everyone, you are not as indispensable and self important as you once may have believed. It is de-stressing just to realize our human input and output quota, to admit (to ourselves) our limits and failings.

We become human. Not superhuman. We become human beings. Not human doings. We take one step back out of the race. We bow out gracefully. Our values change. The fatness of our wallet becomes less important as we become valuable to ourselves. We treat ourselves better. We make time for ourselves.

We allow ourselves to be who we want to be. We stop taking center stage and striving for applause. You have to take your self to task and look at all areas of stress in your life. And change them. This takes time and never really stops.

Now I no longer think I have to call all the shots, I am a better listener, I let others take responsibility, I am less rushed, and I consider others more. I am interested in other people's points of view and will hear them out, I notice the wind in the trees. I am less stressed.

Laugh.
Love. Live.

The effect of happiness will have a great impact on your health. Laughing is a regenerative activity. It is statistically proven, people who are sick, recover quickly and more comprehensively, when they laugh. Great ways to let laughter into your life are joke books and cartoons, comedy movies, anything that gives you a laugh. Always look on the funny side of life. Cut back on the dim and grim channels on TV and tune into laughter. It is the best medicine and that is a scientifically proven fact. The more you laugh out load, the more side-splitting rolling on the floor you can do. The better you feel, the better you become!

Water and sunshine are healing balms. At every opportunity soak in the bath or in the sea. Look for pleasures and pursue them. Make every little thing into a pleasure. It's part of my wellness formula. You know the saying, if God is in the detail, well, that's where you should look.

Give yourself permission to not feel guilty about taking a little time out. It's another step towards feeling in control of your life. Try that one. It's not as easy as it sounds. You will find how stressed you are when you think relaxation is a negative. We have so much guilt attached to not working. We inherently see it as being lazy. Go ahead. Take a break and enjoy it.

The other regenerative activity is love. If you have someone to love, there's a lot of research to say our recovery and life will be far more successful. Touching, feeling, getting physical with a lover, kissing, holding, stroking. Giving and receiving physical comfort and affection is a gift. All these activities create endorphins, the feel good hormones in our body. Everything we do with and for love creates healing in our body. The more we give love, the more we feel loved, the more energy, life force and regenerative power happens inside us. If your living on your own, think about getting a pet. The love of people and animals have tremendous healing properties.

Postscript

In the four years following my diagnosis of Meniere's, I continually challenged myself.

Meniere's was a huge learning curve. I learned to balance with weight bearing exercises and core strength work. I learned to ski, snowboard, surf and windsurf. I increased my fitness, altered my diet, added vitamin and mineral supplements, studied meditation techniques and tried various alternative therapies. I spend time worrying less and loving more. And as I improved my physical health, I made a new life.

Not only do I understand Meniere's as a condition, having experienced life with it; I also understand the lack of understanding and compassion one can find within the social structure, and the subsequent additional damage that situation brings to Meniere's sufferers. In fact, it was an educated man of authority and power, who said to me and I quote "Your Meniere's is a mere inconvenience." His comment caused me and my family serious long term damage that was beyond repair. Until non-sufferers understand Meniere's disease, then sufferers are vulnerable on a physical, mental, emotional level because they may not receive the support necessary to cope.

And worse, people who have Meniere's disease may be taken advantage of. The fact is, there are people in society who are aggressive predators looking to take advantage. These people exist. So be aware and seek as much genuine support as you can. You need it.

Meniere's has allowed other qualities to come forward in my life; compassion; love and the ability for empathy. Without empathy, we are not human.

The miniature cochlea bone, inside the inner ear, is a symbol of how small things can be important. *The Self Help Book For Meniere's Disease* is a small step for me but, as the Astronaut could have said, a small step for this man, but a giant leap for Meniere kind. And if you are reading it, I hope it is a sure and positive step forward for you too. I hope this book and my experience inspire you to find ways to cope with Meniere's. To find new ways to limit symptoms of vertigo. So you can ultimately recover your sense of equilibrium and well-being.

For me, I have made a total recovery, apart from Tinnitus and reduced hearing in one ear. Even that has advantages. When there is a neighborhood party, I don't hear loud music. I sleep like a baby! There are actually some benefits that can come from suffering from illness. You get to know your body, its limitations and unlimited potential.

One Hundred Ways Of Coping With Meniere's

1. Buy a new journal

2. Write down goals

3. Keep track of changes

4. Write down my vitamin regime

5. Start with single vitamin supplements

6. Try Vitamin E and Vitamin C for starters

7. Increase or decrease the dose

8. Extra vitamins to boost my system

9. My daily exercise routine

10. Make a plan

11. Make some goals

12. Get moving

13. Keep moving

14. Do more than you feel like doing

15. Just start walking

16. My daily goal for walking

17. Step by step

18. How far can I go

19. How long are my walks

20. Increase time of walks

21. Increase duration of walks

22. Go further than before

23. Use lamp posts as markers

24. Walk in the morning

25. Walk in the evening

26. Take the stairs

27. Get fighting fit

28. Listen to my body

29. Rest

30. Feel alive

31. Breathe the air

32. Get to the beach

33. Find a patch of sunlight

34. Take a long shower

35. Lie in the bath

36. Do more for me

37. Do more for others

38. Small things count big time

39. Keep up in my daily journal

40. Spend time with friends

41. Phone someone

42. Take photographs

43. Do what I love to do

44. Look after my self

45. Think about me

46. Focus on my needs

47. Increase fitness levels

48. Do daily exercise

49. Small steps matter

50. Enrol in a gym

51. Meet my personal trainer

52. Set a training program together

53. Increase walking

54. Increase workouts

55. Small incremental steps

56. Increase weights

57. My current exercise goal is:

58. When I reach my goal, I'll set another one

59. Get a fitness ball for home

60. Write out an eating plan

61. Try eating 6 small meals a day

62. Cook a recipe I love

63. Be unlimited

64. Throw the salt shaker away

65. Pepper not salt

66. Replace salt with herbs

67. Clean the pantry

68. Throw out salted foods

69. Clear out the fridge

70. Go shopping for low salt items

71. Plant a herb garden

72. What have I cut down on

73. What foods have I eliminated.

74. How have I reduced salt intake

75. My experience of alternative therapies

76. My meditation times

77. Make up a personal healing mantra

78. Write my affirmations down

79. What's working for me

80. How am I feeling

81. What do I want to change

82. Personal challenges

83. My main triggers

84. What are my main stressors

85. What stress have I reduced

86. Have I laughed lately

87. Subscribe to the comedy channel

88. The small stuff. I won't sweat it

89. Get meditation CDs'

90. Love a lot

91. Relax

92. Aromatherapy

93. Small steps count to recovery

94. Book in a massage

95. Go swimming

96. Take time to be in nature

97. Take up a creative activity

98. Make everything I do a step forward

99. Get out more

100. Believe in better health

If I can do it. So can you.

Meniere Man

MENIERE MAN BOOKS

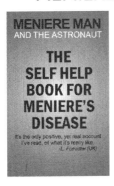

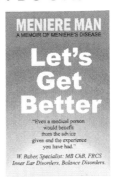

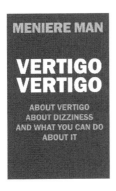

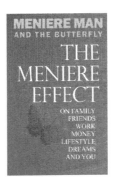

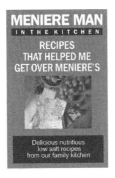

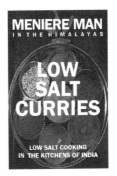

Books By Meniere Man

Let's Get Better:
A Memoir of Meniere's Disease

Let's Get Better CD:
Relaxing & Healing Guided Meditation Voiced by Meniere Man

Vertigo Vertigo:
About Vertigo About Dizziness and What You Can Do About it.

Meniere Man And The Astronaut:
The Self Help Book for Meniere's Disease

Meniere Man And The Butterfly. The Meniere Effect:
How to Minimize the Effect of Meniere's on Family, Money, Lifestyle, Dreams and You.

Meniere Man in the Kitchen:
Lets Get Cooking. Delicious Low Salt Recipes From Our Family Kitchen.

Meniere Man In The Himalayas:
Low Salt Curries. Low Salt Cooking in the Kitchens of India

Meniere's Support Networks And Societies

Meniere's Society (UNITED KINGDOM)
www. menieres.org.uk

Meniere's Society Australia
(AUSTRALIA)info@menieres.org.au

The Meniere's Resource & Information Centre
(AUSTRALIA) www.menieres.org.au

Healthy Hearing & Balance Care (AUSTRALIA)
www.healthyhearing.com.au

Vestibular Disorders association (AUSTRALIA)
www.vestibular .org

The Dizziness and Balance Disorders Centre
(AUSTRALIA)
www.dizzinessbalancedisorders.com

Meniere's Research Fund Inc   (AUSTRALIA)
www.menieresresearch.org.au

Australian Psychological Society APS
(AUSTRALIA) www.psychology.org.au

Meniere's Disease Information Center (USA)
www.menieresinfo.com

Vestibular Disorders Association (USA)
www.vestibular.org

BC Balance and Dizziness Disorders Society
(CANADA) www.balanceand dizziness.org

Hearwell (NEW ZEALAND)
www.hearwell.co.nz

WebMD.
www.webmd.com

National Institute for Health
www.medlineplus.gov

Mindful Living Program
www.mindfullivingprograms.com

Center for Mindfulness
www. umassmed.edu.com

Books
Meniere Man
Recommends

Mindful Way Through Depression.

-By Jon Kabat-Zinn

Full Catastrophe Living.

-By Jon Kabat-Zinn

Mindfulness Based Stress Reduction Workbook.

-By Jon Kabat-Zinn

The Man Who Mistook His Wife for a Hat.

-By Oliver Sacks

Stumbling on Happiness.

-By Daniel Todd Gilbert

Still Alice.

-By Lisa Genova

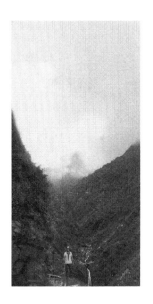

About
Meniere Man

With a smile and a sense of humor, the Author pens himself as Meniere Man, because, as he says, Meniere's disease changed his life dramatically. At the height of his business career and aged just forty-six, he suddenly became acutely ill. He was diagnosed with Meniere's disease. He began to lose all hope that he would fully recover his health. However the full impact of having Meniere's disease was to come later. He lost not only his health, but also his career and financial status as well.

It was his personal spirit and desire to get "back to normal" that turned his life around for the better. He decided that you can't put a limit on anything in life. Rather than letting Meniere's disease get in the way of life, he started to focus on what to do about overcoming Meniere's disease.

With the advice on healing and recovery in his books, anyone reading the advice given, can make simple changes and find a way toward a recovery from Meniere's disease. These days life is different for the Author. He is a fit man who has no symptoms of Meniere's except for tinnitus and hearing loss in one ear. He does not take any medication. All the physical activities he enjoys these days require a high degree of balance: snowboarding, surfing, hiking, windsurfing, weightlifting, and riding a motorbike. All these things he started to do while suffering with Meniere's disease symptoms. Meniere Man believes that if you want to experience a marked improvement in health you can't wait until you feel well to start. You must begin to improve your health immediately, even though you may not feel like it.

The Author is a writer, painter, designer and exhibiting artist. He is married to a Poet and Essayist. They have two adult children. He spends his time writing and painting. He loves the sea, cooking, traveling, nature and the company of family, friends and his beloved Phu Quoc dog.

Additional Information

If you enjoyed this book and you think it could be helpful to others, please leave a review for the book at amazon.com amazon.co.uk or Goodreads. Thank you. This book and other Meniere Man books are available worldwide from international booksellers and local bookstores including Amazon.com, Amazon.co.uk, Barnes & Noble Books. Available in paperback and Kindle.

24238716R00090

Printed in Great Britain
by Amazon